Journey Home

From Cambodia to Canada & Beyond

Rose & Wilson Ngo

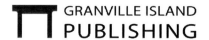

GRANVILLE ISLAND
PUBLISHING

ISBN: 978-1-989467-60-2 (paperback)
ISBN: 978-1-989467-61-9 (ebook)

Editor: Jessica Kaplan
Copy editor: Marianne Ward
Book designer: Jamie Fischer
Map: Jamie Fischer

Granville Island Publishing Ltd.
105 – 1496 Cartwright St.
#14354, Granville Island
Vancouver, BC, Canada, V6H 4J6

604-688-0320 / 1-877-688-0320
info@granvilleislandpublishing.com
www.granvilleislandpublishing.com

Printed in Canada on recycled paper

Dedication

In loving memory of Wilson, my husband and the father of our twins, who asked me to write this for him as soon as possible after his passing. One of his greatest fears was that our twins wouldn't remember their beloved daddy. I know with certainty they will learn how incredible he was through the sharing of his story, and I feel blessed to do this for him.

— Rose

Contents

Author's Note

During our many years together, Wilson and I often spoke about documenting the events his family had endured before finally ending up in Canada. It was evident that this story was important to him, as he regularly shared with me detailed accounts of his family's hardships. He eventually asked me, many years ago now, if I would co-author a book with him. At the time, I told him that I wasn't a writer but that I would help him when I retired. But as we continued to journey through life together, I began jotting down the details and keeping a record of major events as he spoke or wrote about them.

As Wilson's life took a turn for the worse, I asked him what I could do for him. He told me that his biggest regret was not being able to watch his children grow up, to not have them know him or feel how much he truly loved them. He wanted so badly to have a relationship with them. I promised him that I would finish putting together all the stories he had told me so that I could pass it on to our children. They would get to know Wilson through me.

This was the beginnings of my legacy project for Wilson. I knew before I started this project that my late husband was an amazing man, but it was in its creation that I truly saw the depths at which his life impacted those around him. In the process of interviewing his family members and friends to solidify details, I was fortunate to capture memories that have since become lost, as two of his aunts have succumbed to varying degrees of dementia. What a true blessing it has been for me to document Wilson's life, and to now share it with you and with our children.

— *Rose*

Prologue

It is so clear to me now that God has a purpose for each of us—for me. My walk with the Lord has been a shaky one. But regardless of my attitude toward Him, God has always been there in the background to catch me when I fall. He has our back … always.

A non-spiritual person might classify my life as one of chance and coincidence, but a person of faith might say it was nothing short of miraculous. In reflecting upon the events of my life, I cannot deny the existence of God. I am no more special than any other human being. In fact, following the Christian life doesn't mean everything is fair or easy. It is in the tough times that we see who we truly are and who is left standing with us until the bitter end.

— Wilson

1

Who Exactly Am I?

I am Wilson—a child of God. God wasn't always at the forefront of my mind. In fact, for most of my life I was either angry with Him or trying to ignore Him. When people look at me, they often see my loving wife, a cute set of young twins, my close relationship with siblings and parents, a beautiful house, a successful career and many friends. But what they don't see is the struggle I endured for these things.

So ... who exactly am I? What makes me who I am? Do the things I do and the choices I make really matter? These are the questions I have asked myself countless times throughout my life, and they were finally answered at its end.

My parents named me well. My Chinese name, 吳美興, means 'Beautiful Happiness', and I lived up to my name—often smiling and joking around, even when I was hurting inside. I often told my wife, Rose, how I was a "simple man with simple needs." But how far from the truth that was, as nothing about my life has been simple. Every seemingly simple question has a complicated answer.

I was born in Phnom Penh, Cambodia, but my legal documents state otherwise. A full understanding of this requires an account of my genealogy. (Although this part may seem boring, it is instrumental to understanding my story, much like how the book of Genesis shows how Jesus is connected to Adam.)

My paternal grandfather, 吳金貢, was 50 percent Cambodian and 50 percent Chinese (from Chaozhou). The second eldest of five children, he was born in Cambodia but was sent to China at age nine to live with his father's grandmother and her family, to have a chance at a 'better' life and to ensure the continuation of the family bloodline. Without a son who would go on to marry and have children, the family tree would have ended, bringing shame and pity to the family. This was especially important since he was now the only surviving son. His two elder brothers had recently died from illness, leaving behind my grandfather and his two sisters.

In China, my grandfather worked as a messenger boy until my great-great-grandfather was able to buy three shops, a fish farm and a home for the entire family to live in. At seventeen, my grandfather had an arranged marriage to a local Chinese woman (from Chaozhou), who was then sixteen. My grandma, 林尖, was the village beauty. My grandfather, on the other hand, was not very handsome. But because of his great-grandfather, he was quite wealthy.

Shortly after my grandparents were married, my grandma had two sons, both of whom died shortly after birth. Soon my aunt, 吳林專, was born, closely followed by my father, Ngo Van Liem, 吳培林, who was born at the end of the Second World War, in 1945. A year later, China suffered a severe famine, and my grandfather bought four boat tickets and moved his immediate family back to where he had been born, a village named Svaay Rieng in Cambodia. After moving to Cambodia, my grandmother gave birth to her second daughter, my father's younger sister, who ended up contracting a virus that killed her shortly after her first birthday.

Although my grandfather had been a great businessman in China, things were different in Cambodia, and he ended up providing for his family by becoming the town baker. Unfortunately, my father never picked up a skill or talent for baking. Instead, he completed secondary school and qualified to become a teacher. However, his deepest desire was to become a successful businessman, as his father had been in China.

My mother, Tran Tu Nguyet, was born in Svaay Rieng, Cambodia, in 1947. She was the eldest child and had four sisters. Her grandfather, whose surname was Wong, was 100 percent Chinese, and her grandmother was 75 percent Vietnamese and 25 percent Cambodian. My mother's mother, who was 50 percent Chinese, 38 percent Vietnamese and 12 percent Cambodian, married a man whose surname was Tran and who was 100 percent Chinese. Put simply, my mother was approximately 20 percent Vietnamese, 5 percent Cambodian and 75 percent Chinese (from Chaozhou with Wong/

Tran family roots), and my father was 25 percent Cambodian and 75 percent Chinese. (Our various ethnic backgrounds are intentionally mentioned, not just as fun facts, but more importantly, to show how God would use our family roots to save us.)

My mother completed her education at a grade-four level in Mandarin, and when she was eighteen years old, it was arranged for her to marry my father, who was then twenty. It was customary at that time for parents to find partners for their children. Mostly, these marriages were established to ensure financial security and reputation. In my parents' case, neither party was particularly thrilled about the arrangement, especially since my mother had her eyes set on another man, one who also happened to be interested in her. To boot, my father, a flirtatious and handsome young man, clearly wasn't ready to settle down. However, to honour tradition and appease their families, my parents chose to make the marriage work. Time and again, they would prove that with hard work and determination, they could overcome any obstacle. It is through their modelling that I have been able to embody this notion of 'grit' that is rooted in who I am.

Shortly after their wedding on August 6, 1964, my father started a business fixing bikes and selling tires. Three years later, he closed up shop and began to sell ceramics instead. By 1970, there was a considerable amount of civil and social unrest in Cambodia as the Khmer Rouge slowly infiltrated the political landscape.

The Khmer Rouge was an extremist communist movement and totalitarian regime within Cambodia led by the military leader—and eventual prime minister—Pol Pot. Among other aims, the regime intended to wipe out all traces of Western influences in Cambodia and is considered to have been one of the most brutal Marxist governments in the twentieth century. In response to the increasing power and threat of the Khmer Rouge, my parents, along with my grandparents and aunts, sold their home and business and moved to the capital city of Phnom Penh. By this point, my mother had given birth to three children: my two older sisters and my brother.

For the next two years in Phnom Penh, my parents invested in their trading business, selling a multitude of household products. As the country was embroiled in civil war, complete with bombings in 1973, my paternal grandfather had a stroke and passed away. Six months later, as political tensions continued to worsen in Cambodia, I was born on January 16, 1974.

At the time of my birth, there was a lot of negative talk about how difficult life would become under the Khmer Rouge due to their grass-roots ideology, which was to "cleanse, purify and rebuild Cambodia." They wished to overthrow the capitalist government and return to a simple farming-based socialist regime. Their hate for Westerners was so severe that they had made it a practice to capture and imprison educated adult Cambodians so that future generations would not be influenced with Western ideals. Adults who would not 'bow down' to the new political regime would be reeducated. Children were forced to become cold killers and soldiers.

With foreign government officials leaving Cambodia, my parents knew that we could not stay in our mother country any longer. Our family had to leave, especially since we were not 'pure' Cambodians. The Khmer Rouge considered us 'half-bloods' or 'mutts'. If we had stayed, we would have stained the purity of their new Cambodia; therefore, we would have been killed. Our destination now was Vietnam—by foot.

2

Exodus from the Killing Fields: Journey to Vietnam

Our journey to Vietnam began on March 20, 1975. We left our home and family business behind. Vietnam was not only the obvious choice geographically, but more so because my mother had some close relatives there who were willing to help support and settle us while we transitioned to our new home in a foreign country. However, from a political standpoint, the Chinese were considered an enemy of Vietnam because China had supported the South during the Vietnam War. To ensure that Cambodia maintained peace with its neighbour, Khmer Rouge soldiers were instructed to capture anyone attempting to cross the Vietnamese–Cambodian border who was of Chinese ancestry.

Since we were part Chinese, it was important that we kept this part of our identity a secret. If we disclosed our full identity at the border, at best we would not be allowed to enter Vietnam, and at worst, we would be pulled aside by the Khmer Rouge.

To complicate things further, my mother was nine months pregnant with my youngest sister during our exodus. Our family unit consisted of my pregnant mother (aged twenty-eight), my father (aged thirty), my three sisters (aged four, six and ten), my eight-year-old brother and fifteen-month-old me. We travelled with our extended family, which included my four aunts, my maternal grandparents (Grandma and Grandpa Tran) and paternal grandmother (Grandma Ngo).

Our currency, the Cambodian riel, was now worthless—my mother later told me that soldiers were taking bills in large barrels from the banks and throwing them out onto the streets—and the Khmer Rouge wanted to rule without the use of a national currency. Luckily, my parents had converted their monetary assets before the riel's devaluation. We were literally leaving Cambodia with $1,000 USD and some gold taels, a unit of weight for Chinese currency, in our pockets to use as seed money for starting over in Vietnam. We also took things of value that we could carry, like rice, skim milk powder (for me), jewellery and anything else that we could use for bartering. As we were making preparations to leave, Grandma Tran instructed my second aunt to purchase a large quantity of sewing needles and two large spools of white and black thread.

We loaded up our car, a light-blue 1970s French import, with heavy items like rice, cooking pots and my pregnant mother. Despite having a car, everyone walked, including my grandparents. At the beginning of our trek, my father would slowly drive the car alongside us as we walked. We were often moving so slowly that we were aggravated by the fumes and heat from the car exhaust. Eventually, the car ran out of gas, and my grandparents enlisted all able-bodied family members, mainly my four aunts, to help push the car as we made our walk to freedom.

Even without gasoline, our family relied on our car as not only a storage vessel, but also as shelter from the intermittent periods of wind and rain. When a downpour hit, my pregnant mom, me, my elderly grandparents and any other sibling who could fit, all huddled inside the car while the others sought shelter under a nearby tree or tarp.

We were not the only people leaving Phnom Penh. It has been reported that over the course of April 1975, nearly two million people evacuated the city. As did many others, we travelled as a group alongside five other families, making us twenty-one people in total. There was no apparent leader in our group, and no one had a map to guide us. We just knew we had to head south to get to Vietnam. Our group was fortunate in that God blessed us with a skilled nurse who would be instrumental in helping deliver my youngest sister into this world.

The geographic distance from Phnom Penh to the Vietnam border is approximately 120 kilometres. Every day, after packing our camp from the night before, we were limited to walking from two o'clock to five o'clock, due to the extreme heat, with temperatures reaching into

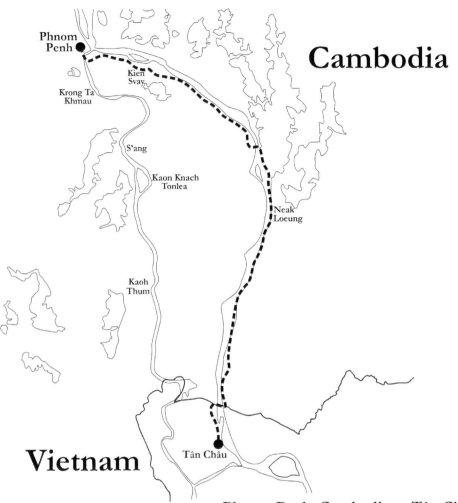

Phnom Penh, Cambodia to Tân Châu,
An Giang Province, Vietnam by foot

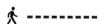

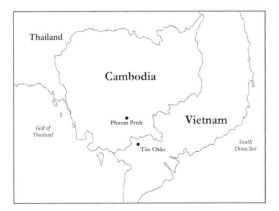

the mid to high thirties (Celsius), and the pitch-black night that would envelope us shortly after five o'clock. Consequently, we could only cover a few kilometres a day due to the size of the group and the ages within our multifamily unit, coupled with the fact that we were pushing a car. We were not the only family struggling to make this journey, and we saw many dead bodies along the sides of the roads, both young and old. It was not out of the ordinary to find people scavenging the remains, looking for food, jewellery or other items of value.

Because the Cambodian government was anxious for us to exit the country in a timely fashion, Khmer Rouge soldiers were stationed at many village posts situated along all major routes heading out of Cambodia, monitoring our exodus. We were herded in and out of villages like cattle each day. No one dared to cross any of these soldiers; they were young and revelled in their power to instill fear in others. If anyone disrespected or stepped out of line—so much as even raised their voice when speaking to a Khmer Rouge soldier—he or she would be executed on the spot. Villagers were allowed to trade goods with us, but they were prohibited from taking us into their homes. Any such action would have led to extreme punishment or execution, done to ensure that the minds of 'pure-bred Cambodian' villagers would not become corrupted or tainted by people like us—'mutt-like' city dwellers.

The Cambodia my family knew and loved was gone. It had been replaced by a military regime, and the people's voice would no longer be heard. Our opinions no longer mattered. This was the end of what little democracy Cambodia had. Our lives were now at the mercy of young, power-hungry, trigger-happy, brainwashed soldiers. This only fuelled and strengthened our need and will to leave behind our beloved homeland.

Although we had some US currency and gold, it was actually my aunt's three hundred sewing needles and two giant spools of thread that would ensure we made it out of Cambodia alive. At each major stop we made, we bartered and traded for rice, fish, poultry and powdered milk. Sometimes, a single sewing needle could be traded for a few pounds of fish or a few kilos of yams, or a shirt for two chickens. At one point, we even traded a stereo for fifteen chickens!

In retrospect, God was gracious in that we were travelling during Cambodia's hot and dry season. Had it been during the monsoon season, our trek would have been longer, as roads would have been flooded, forcing us to cover less ground each day. However, even in this dry season we endured the inconvenience of short 'mango' showers in the afternoons.

These afternoon showers forced our walking to a halt as we had to seek refuge in our car or under nearby trees. Once the showers passed, we would resume our trek. Despite travelling in the midst of a tropical jungle teaming with natural wildlife, we rarely saw snakes or other animals because we travelled in such large groups and close to dirt roads.

Every day around five o'clock, we would set up 'camp' wherever we were, often at the side of the road. We would hang a tarp between nearby trees under which the adults would sleep, while my youngest siblings, my mother and I slept in the car. I cannot imagine how scared, desperate and lost my parents must have felt during this exodus. My father told me that we even slept in a cemetery one night. They were clinging to hope—a hope that they could be free to have a better life, not just for themselves but for us, their children. What faith, love and courage they had!

Because my mother was nine months pregnant, it was Grandma Ngo who carried me piggyback most of the time. (She was relatively healthy compared to my other grandma. Grandma Tran had a weak heart, and the stress of this journey proved hard on both her mind and her body. She had to take frequent breaks when walking and often needed to ride in the car next to my mother. The notion of having to leave behind all she knew made her anxious and fearful.) My aunts told me that they frequently caught Grandma Ngo sighing, commenting on how heavy I was. All my mother could do was smile, recognizing she was in no position to carry me.

I was a growing toddler and was naturally hungry quite often. In the times when we had no access to powdered milk, I cried incessantly for food. To stop me from crying, my mother fed me sugared water or watered-down congee, a rice soup. As a parent myself now, I would do anything to soothe and comfort my children and address their physical needs, so I can appreciate how utterly helpless and heartbroken my mother must have felt to see me cry for food when we didn't have any and to know there was little she could do to change that reality.

Although we loved the convenience of having our car, without enough food to fuel our bodies, my aunts became too weak to push the vehicle. Thus, my dad decided that we needed to remove the engine from the car to reduce its weight. At one of the next villages, he borrowed some tools and with the help of family members, he successfully removed and discarded the engine, and our car instantly became lighter. But about halfway to Vietnam, as we followed the Mekong River south, the roads became narrow dirt trails. We would now have to abandon our car—our comfort and safety. Saying goodbye was bittersweet. On the one hand, it meant we were closer to reaching our destination, but on the other, it now meant there was no turning back.

Every morning, my father and other able-bodied members in our group foraged for food at nearby abandoned farms. We often found unharvested vegetables and even poultry. One time we even managed to catch a pig, which we then butchered, salt cured and fried, rendering the fat to store for future use as cooking oil. In sharing this memory with me, my second aunt smiled as she recalled savouring the bits of deep-fried pig skin and meat that she snacked on during our walk or breaks.

During one of our scavenges, we found an ox cart. It was truly heaven-sent as walking, now without our car, was difficult for my very pregnant mother, me, my siblings and my grandparents. With the ox cart, stronger members in our group could now push tired members instead of us stopping altogether. This way, we could still press onward.

Because we travelled along the river or nearby lakes, we collected water as needed and boiled it before drinking. When we were lucky, we caught fish or shellfish. Most importantly, we gathered wood, for without it we had no fire with which to cook the rice. In truth, however, only my pregnant mother and elderly grandparents ate rice; the rest of us lived off of watered-down congee.

Unbeknownst to us, on Thursday, April 17, 1975, after seizing Phnom Penh, the Khmer Rouge decreed they would "rebuild Cambodia" and, at gunpoint, required everyone to evacuate the city and head toward neighbouring villages. It was a good thing that God had prompted us to start our trek almost a month earlier. Had we stayed, we would likely have been enslaved or executed.

My sister was born on Sunday, April 20, 1975, in an abandoned house in a timber yard en route to Vietnam. Luckily, my mother had previous experience with two home deliveries, and we had the expertise of a nurse in our travel group. That night, we had a feast in celebration of my sister's birth. We found a pig and some ducks and scavenged for vegetables at neighbouring farms. My family believed that my sister's birth was a sign that change was coming, drawing in new positive energy and forecasting a prosperous future. Hence, they named her My Binh, 吳美平, which means 'Beautiful Peace'.

Perhaps it was the birth of my sister, or maybe it was the instinctive knowledge that we were closer to Vietnam that allowed my family to experience a resurgence of energy and hope which allowed us to cover more ground.

Foreshadowing a change, at one of our next stops, a Khmer Rouge soldier overheard my grandfather speaking Chinese to another group of travellers. (Up until this point, we had all been careful to limit any needless chatter.) In hearing my grandfather speak Chinese, the Khmer Rouge soldier immediately grabbed him from our campsite and forced him into a small boat bound for the military base across the river. Grandpa Tran was being detained.

My whole family was devastated; all the women—my aunts, mother and grandmothers—were crying and wailing with despair: "We have come so far and are only days away from reaching Vietnam. How can this be happening?" My second aunt knew instinctively that she would never see her father again if we didn't get him back from the Khmer Rouge soldiers as soon as possible. I can only explain her sudden courage and wisdom as coming from God, for she immediately jumped into action, telling the rest of our family, "You need to continue on the journey to Vietnam. Don't wait for me and Dad. I'm going to get him back. I can't leave him behind. I will find you, and we will rejoin you."

She found someone paddling a small boat who was willing to take her across the river to the military base. She offered the paddler some money, but to her surprise, he replied, "Money is of no use here. You keep it." This boatman must have been amazed at what my aunt was willing to do to save her father. When they docked and were met by high-ranking military officials, my aunt began weeping, begging and pleading for the safe return of her father. How utterly heroic and insane my aunt was!

"General, my father is not Chinese but Cambodian. He only knows how to speak Chinese because his grandpa was Chinese. It is only through his ancestral roots that he speaks Chinese. My father married my mother—a Vietnamese woman. My mother and my sisters are truly Cambodian, with Vietnamese and Chinese roots. Please do not take my father. We need him. He is our anchor. We will not survive without him. My mother is very sick. My older sister just gave birth a few days ago. We have been travelling for one month already. We are weak and starving. We have nothing left to eat. If you can, please, please, let my father go… and spare us some rice."

The military official must have been moved by my aunt's persistence and bravery, because in a miraculous act that I can only see as God's mercy, the official not only allowed both my aunt and Grandpa Tran to return to the other side of the river, but also gifted her with a bag of rice. When the family saw both of them returning there was an ecstatic celebration complete with sobs of relief and yelps of joy. Everyone commended my second aunt for her quick, cunning action and extreme bravery.

It was now Wednesday, April 30, 1975. We had left Phnom Penh forty days earlier and were now moments from arriving in Tân Châu, a Vietnamese city just on the outskirts of the Cambodia/Vietnam border. There were crowds of people—hundreds, perhaps even thousands— standing on the shoreline awaiting their turn to ride across the river in small boats to Tân Châu, to freedom.

The boarding process was chaotic, and my second aunt took the opportunity for the family to save some money while ensuring we all were able to board. Money was tight, and we would need what little we had to provide for ourselves in Vietnam. During the boarding process, my eldest siblings waited just next to the shuttle boat with their heads submerged underwater or hid themselves among the adults who were also waiting to board.

Once everyone was seated on the small boat, the lady who was re- sponsible for collecting money made a beeline for my second aunt and said, "Sister, you didn't pay enough." Because Cambodian currency was worthless under this new military, Communist regime, transactions were made using gold. It was obvious that these boat operators didn't have ex- perience handling gold currency and were easily confused with currency conversion. My second aunt, who had learned to speak Vietnamese with a Viet Cong accent due to her previous business dealings with this powerful and influential group, led the shuttle boat operators to believe she was a person of power—a Viet Cong official working in Cambodia, returning home—and they didn't dare mess with her.

She raised her voice and declared, "How dare you! I am a member of the Viet Cong. Are you questioning my authority and honesty? I clearly gave you enough. You are the one who is mistaken! The Viet Cong are expecting my return. If you do not want any trouble, you will leave me be." The lady from the boat team complied, clearly shaken. She did not want any repercussions from messing with members of the Viet Cong. My second aunt, though nervous as hell on the inside, did not break out of character. God's veil of protection was clearly upon our family.

Our shuttle boat docked a short distance from the border. We walked to the crossing where we stated that we were Vietnamese foreigners seeking refuge in Vietnam. Because we spoke the language and the border guards knew there would be a need for more farmers in the country's new socialist regime, we were granted entry. This is when my father formally changed the spelling of our Chinese surname to the Vietnamese phonetic equivalent, Ngo.

Because droves of us were entering Vietnam from Cambodia, the Vietnamese government housed us in an empty school in Tân Châu for three nights while the officials finished our paperwork. We converted what was left of our gold to Vietnamese currency, the Vietnamese dong. Once our papers were processed, we purchased train tickets to Saigon to stay with one of Grandma Tran's sisters.

In retelling this story, my father often reflected on the fear he felt during this time. He remembered asking himself multiple times a day during our exodus if we'd ever make it out of Cambodia alive, but he never regretted his decision to leave. Little did he know at the time that children in Cambodia were brainwashed to become soldiers of the state—cold killers—and that educated adults would be forced into agricultural labour. Any non-compliance resulted in immediate execution, as evident in the mass graves scattered throughout Cambodia.

These years under the Khmer Rouge would prove to be a dark chapter in Cambodian history. Historians at Yale University estimate a staggering figure of 1 to 3.5 million Cambodians were killed in the name of genocide. These deaths were the result of executions, starvation, disease and accidental death by land mines buried during the civil war. This was a devastating human atrocity.

In my own reflection of this event, I now know that it was not merely my family's determination and strong desire to survive but God's will and grace that ensured we *all* made it to Vietnam. How could I deny that God's hand was there, opening a window whenever a door slammed shut? God had provided all that we needed to survive. Although we were made to feel 'dirty' and unwanted by the Khmer Rouge because we were not 'pure' Cambodians, it was this very impurity that ensured we had a way out.

God's plan ensured that we could cross into Vietnam because of our cultural heritage and relatives. We could have easily suffered a gruelling life of pain or a violent death in Cambodia. But we didn't. And although Grandpa Tran's Chinese did get us into trouble, it would be our very same Chinese heritage that would eventually ensure our passage to Canada.

3

The Great Escape:
From Vietnam to Thailand by Boat

Although we were ecstatic about arriving safely in Vietnam, our enthusiasm was bittersweet. Coincidentally, we had arrived at the Vietnam–Cambodia border just as the country officially ended its twenty-year civil war, on April 30, 1975. South Vietnam had fallen with the capture of its capital, Saigon. Acting President, General Duong Van Minh and his cabinet would surrender unconditionally in the Independence Palace in Saigon. The Vietnamese border guards were surprisingly nice to us, as this day signified the official ascension of the Communist party. It was the dawn of a new regime, with Saigon renamed Ho Chi Minh City, after the Vietnamese Workers' Party leader. We had fled from one Communist country only to find ourselves in another.

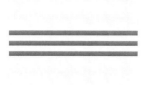 

Left: Pre-war South Vietnam flag   Right: Postwar/current-day Vietnam flag

The next few months in Saigon were extremely difficult. Although we were appreciative of my mom's cousin's hospitality, she herself was living with serious hardships. The home was small and impoverished. Rainwater leaked into the living quarters through multiple holes in the tin roof, and during heavy rains, the nearby riverbank would flood the house. To ensure we and our few belongings stayed relatively dry, we draped a tarp over the roof and slept on the floor. However, there was only enough room for our family of fifteen to sleep sitting up. It was these poor living conditions that forced my aunts and parents to quickly find work.

There was no shortage of jobs in Saigon. My parents started a small business selling and fixing bikes, which they did for about two years, and then they sold car tires for another two. My second aunt sold fabric in a local market, while another two of my aunts illegally sold medications on the streets. According to my third aunt, there were no operating pharmacies due to the formation of the new government regime. Medication was only administered by public health officials and could not be purchased. Hence, pain relief pills were in demand and easy to sell. When everyone was at work, my older siblings attended school while my grandparents babysat me and my younger sister.

With all adults working, we were soon able to purchase a small one-storey house for 3.5 taels, also called cây, lạng or lượng. One tael is equivalent to 37.5 grams or 1.3 ounces of gold. Based on today's gold market (approximately $1,825 US per ounce, as of July 2021), our family paid about US$8,300 for this house. Although it was only the size of a small living room by today's North American standards, it was a huge improvement from where we had been staying. It accommodated the fifteen of us: my parents, four aunts, two grandmothers, one grandfather and the six children. To ensure there was enough room for all of us to sleep properly, my Grandpa Tran built a small loft.

As we slowly found a new rhythm for our lives, we also found joy in our moments together. My parents' shop was about 15 km from where we lived, and in the beginning, they took a bus to work. But as they earned more money, they purchased a motorbike to use as their means of travel. Grandpa Tran cooked and delivered hot lunch to my parents every day, updating them as to how my younger sister and I were doing at home.

Communication between my parents and grandpa became especially important during this time. From 1966 to 1977, there was a global effort to eradicate smallpox that required everyone to be vaccinated, and my younger sister, only one year old at the time, had complications resulting from her vaccination. The needle the nurse had used was dirty, and my sister contracted necrotizing fasciitis, a flesh-eating disease caused by Streptococcus bacteria. A portion of her torso had to be surgically removed. Necrotizing fasciitis is rarely seen in children, and death can be imminent—within twelve to twenty-four hours. Because this was an error on the part of the government-mandated vaccination program, the hospital covered all costs to treat my sister. Here was yet another example of God's grace and hand upon our family. She could have easily died or lost a limb, but that was not a part of God's plan for her life.

In visiting my parents at lunch, Grandpa Tran would also share tales of my bad behaviour. My father had envisioned us emigrating to France because he had a relative there who was willing to sponsor our family. Therefore, it made sense that my younger sister and I attend a private French preschool. But when I wasn't in school, my mischievous side took over. Grandpa Tran would tell my parents of how he would frequently find me acting 'nonchalant', with cuts on my body or blood on my shirt, often the result of fights with the neighbour kids, sometimes fights that were three against my one. I would even brag to Grandpa Tran that the blood on my clothing wasn't mine!

I was told later that when I wasn't in a fight, I was sometimes found sleeping by a lamp post on the side of the street. As a result, Grandpa Tran often had to spend time looking for me, so much so that neighbours eventually got into the routine of reporting to my grandfather where I was. Once I was found, Grandpa Tran would either carry me home fast asleep or stop the village brawl to take me home.

My older brother was often responsible for babysitting me when my grandparents needed a break. He was obsessed with watching rooster fights, and on one occasion, there was a special fight in the neighbouring town when it was his turn to watch me. My brother decided to take me with him by bus to watch this rooster fight, and when my grandfather got wind of where we had gone, he quickly informed my father, who was so upset that he left work early to look for the both of us.

As time moved on, my parents' business flourished. Under normal circumstances, this would have been excellent news, but the political climate of Vietnam was changing. For the first few years after the North took power, private businesses appeared to resume operations as before. But soon the government became adamant about eradicating these businesses that were not in alignment with their ideological and political goals as a Communist state. Hence, private ownership of land and businesses would no longer be allowed.

There were rumours that the Chinese government was planning to retaliate against Vietnam for the persecution of ethnic Chinese nationals, and they also didn't like that Vietnam was occupying Cambodia at the time. This conflict would later be known as the Sino-Vietnamese War. Because many businesses, such as ours, were owned by Sino-Vietnamese, meaning Vietnamese of Chinese descent, we all now had a target on our backs. And since Sino-Vietnamese people controlled much of the trade in southern Vietnam, the Vietnamese government perceived our people as a threat to their political regime. Consequently, the government increased taxes and levies, restricted trade and, in some instances, even confiscated Sino-Vietnamese businesses. There was no doubt in the minds of many that the Vietnamese government had orchestrated this racial divide to 'encourage' people of Chinese-Vietnamese descent to leave the country.

Political and economic conditions in Vietnam had made it so that if you had assets, fleeing seemed the best and only solution. At first, the government put measures in place for us to leave Vietnam both legally and voluntarily, and so my father, along with a group of his business friends, invested money to build a lavish ship capable of housing one thousand people! This ship was to be our ticket out of Vietnam. We were going to leave the country in luxury. Unfortunately, the quick buildup of resentment against the Sino-Vietnamese led the Vietnamese government to rescind their offer of a legal and voluntary emigration, and the ship itself was eventually confiscated.

Meanwhile, the Socialist Republic of Vietnam, in many ways similar to the Khmer Rouge, wanted everyone who had been associated with the previous republican regime in the south to participate in a re-education camp, which included torture, starvation, sickness and hard labour. Nearly a million city dwellers were made to 'voluntarily' clear jungles for agricultural land. Due to lack of trade and inexperienced farmers, starvation was inevitable. For my parents, this was déjà vu. They had only fled Cambodia just a few years prior.

For many, Vietnam was no longer a safe place, and some began to find illegal means to leave the country—mostly by boat. The first 'boat people' fled Vietnam in December 1977. Toward the end of 1978, my father and aunties collectively decided to 'secretly' seek refuge in another country. We did not have the time to wait for the paperwork required for my father's relative to legally sponsor us in France. To ensure the success of our exodus, it was important that the Vietnamese government not know our plan. Destination options included China, Malaysia, Thailand and Hong Kong.

Thailand proved to be our best bet, not only because it was closest to us geographically, which made sense when travelling with young children, but more importantly because of a family connection. My father had a cousin who owned and operated fishing boats and who was now illegally smuggling people from the capital city to a boat waiting in international waters which would then take them the rest of the way to Thailand. This is how my family chose to escape. My second aunt also had connections to an illegal 'smuggling' boat due to her previous relationships with Viet Cong members, but my father's family connection ultimately trumped the non-family one and even resulted in a 'family discount' for us.

It was clear, even at the time, that government officials were profiting from this massive illegal exodus of their fellow countrymen. Even with a family discount, my father paid twenty-seven taels of gold for our family to leave by boat, five taels per adult and two per child. (In today's market, he paid the equivalent of US$65,000!) My aunts were charged the regular rate of seven taels per adult. To people desperate to leave a developing country, those prices were astronomical—it was highway robbery!

It was decided that my third aunt would leave first, one month earlier than the rest of us. She would be our 'guinea pig' and pave the way for us. Because long-distance calls were expensive, she told us that she would send a telegraph message from Thailand to let us know she had made it there safely and to give us pointers on what to expect from the voyage. We knew that the trip would take about one week, so we waited to hear back from her. Unfortunately, we never did.

One month later, when it was our turn to leave, we were still holding out hope of reuniting with my third aunt when we arrived in Thailand. My parents, paternal grandmother, five siblings, fourth aunt and my mother's cousin all set out for the 500 km boat trip across the Gulf of Thailand. My mother recalls us leaving sometime in May 1980.

Because what we were doing was illegal, we had to be hidden. At 3:00 a.m., in the dark and quiet of night, we boarded a small fishing boat and lay under the planks where caught fish were stored. All eleven of us were packed like sardines for the four-hour ride to the bigger boat awaiting us in international waters. My father told us that until we were in international waters, we could be captured and sent back to Vietnam, so we were exceptionally quiet. As we lay quietly, tightly packed under the floorboards, we dreamed of our freedom. We were only a boat ride away from Communist Vietnam, but we were also about to be subjected to unforeseen consequences of our quest for a life of choice and independence.

Although we were happy to be released from the confines of the first boat's small quarters, we were shocked to see that the 'larger' boat, was not, in fact, much larger than the one we had just been on. Even more alarmingly, there were to be one hundred passengers on this second boat, which was originally designed for river travel and was now manned by a local captain, sailing the open seas. There was a definite sense of camaraderie amongst us, as we all hoped for the same thing—safe passage to Thailand.

We quickly boarded and settled into a section on this second boat. The captain reminded us that we were to only have 'essentials' with us, basically only the food we could carry and the clothing we were wearing. There wasn't enough room for excess baggage; we were already over-weight and over capacity. This wasn't a holiday cruise ship but rather a boatload of refugees heading to another country.

Prior to leaving Vietnam, my mother, in her brilliance, had Grandpa Tran drill multiple holes into an old wooden slipper. She had stuffed gold jewellery, some US currency and a diamond into its heels and used this as an inconspicuous storage vessel. Who would think to steal an old pair of wooden slippers? Only my parents knew the value that those shoes carried. My mother figured the fewer the people who knew about it, the safer our family treasure would be.

Imagine the chaos on this medium-sized fishing boat—one hundred bodies, one deck and no source of cover in the middle of the open ocean. My mother delegated child-tending responsibilities to different family members while she tended to me (almost six) and my youngest sister (who was then four). My eight-year-old sister was to be cared for by my mother's cousin, while my father saw to the needs of his mother, Grandma Ngo.

When the captain made the announcement to toss excess baggage, there was a mad rush of people throwing things they didn't need over-board. That's when Grandma Ngo found the old pair of wooden slippers and thought, "How silly! Why would my daughter-in-law pack this? How vain to think you would need a second pair of shoes."

My mother recalls a pit forming in her stomach later that day when she couldn't find the bag her shoes had been in. However, she didn't dare make a fuss when she couldn't find the bag, as she didn't want to draw attention to herself or to the value of what was in those shoes. She also didn't dare accuse her mother-in-law of throwing the shoes into the ocean, along with our small fortune. In the grand scheme of things, my mother knew that we would be fortunate just to make it to shore, even if we would literally have nothing except the clothes we were wearing.

If being exposed to wind, rain, turbulence and extreme heat and being stuffed like sardines on a boat weren't enough, try topping that off with boredom, especially for a child like me. There was nothing to do or see, as we rarely saw any other boats around us. The extreme heat made us feel exhausted, and we really had nothing to eat. We rationed and nibbled on dry snacks, since we had no means of cooking. At night it was pitch-black, so we just tried to sleep.

Pirates were known to wait in international waters, often attacking a few days after boats left Vietnam. They took advantage of the fact that passengers would be weak from excessive heat exposure and lack of food. They knew these boats were full of desperate, unarmed people, many of whom were women and children. They also knew many of these people were rich enough to pay for an illegal ride out of their home country. In 1981, the UN High Commissioner for Refugees estimated that 77 percent of the boats leaving Vietnam during this period were attacked by pirates.

While we had all heard the stories, none of us had actually packed knives or guns with which to defend ourselves. Even if we had wanted to bring aboard a weapon, it would have been next to impossible with the Vietnamese government's restrictions and sanctions on firearms—weapons were only available to those in the military. We were on this boat with no protection. We just had to pray that we wouldn't encounter any pirates.

Approximately two days after we boarded the second boat, a large Thai fishing boat approached us early in the morning. Recognizing we were refugees, they demanded that we 'voluntarily' hand over our valuables. Hearing a few of us speak Chinese, they communicated with us in the same dialect. These pirates did not board our ship, nor did we see them pull out firearms, but they did wield knives as they called us forward in small groups to ask us for items like jewellery, in particular gold jewellery, and useful tools, like our boat's compass. Because we were exhausted and wanted no trouble, we complied. This raid lasted less than two hours.

We were fortunate in that there had been no violence and that they had not taken our clothes. In fact, they had given us water, buns and some ice 'in exchange' for our valuables. Some on the boat speculated that they showed us kindness because of our common Chinese roots, yet another blessing through God's providence. We all heaved a great sigh of relief as we watched the pirates sail away. But this relief was short-lived. We were left with a great deal of angst since they had taken our compass—we were now lost at sea.

Our captain was devastated and afraid to die at sea. In desperation, he gathered us together and said, "Comrades, we have nothing, not even a compass! We are lost. We must turn back. I can get us home. We need to head back to Vietnam or we will die out here." There was pushback from a group of outraged men who told the captain in no uncertain terms that going back to Vietnam was not an option.

Later that evening, the captain had an upset stomach. He asked my dad to keep watch and ensure that the ship stayed its course. We heard a loud noise and the sound of something heavy dropping into the water. After a while, my dad, still at the helm, started asking others who were awake if they had seen the captain. No one had. The next morning, a young man stepped forward and told us that he was an ex-marine and knew how to steer our boat. He explained that the captain had accidentally fallen in the water and that it had been too dark for anyone to save him.

After a day of smooth sailing, things took a turn for the worse. Early the next morning, a Thai boat was quickly coming toward us. My aunt and my mother's cousin described this group of experienced and cruel pirates as "ugly" and "aggressive." They flashed their guns and began screaming at us when they were within hearing distance. Within a matter of minutes, a few of them boarded our boat and without speaking, sense-lessly started to use stingray tails to whip the first man they saw. They kept brutally whipping him until all we could focus on was the sight of blood and the cries of pain. In one action, these pirates had instantly instilled fear in the ninety-nine of us left onboard the boat.

Once they had our attention, all the remaining men were told to either jump overboard or be kicked into the water. Because my third sister was under the direct care of my mother's cousin, she followed him as he jumped into the water. She was only eight years old. My mother's cousin quickly tried to hoist her back into the boat. With what can only be explained as a sudden act of grace, one of the pirates saw my sister and pulled her out of the water and back onto the boat to join the rest of the women and children. Had she been left to tread water, she likely would have died.

The men were forced to tread water by the side of the boat and were forbidden to cling to the side of the vessel. Any who moved too close were physically pushed away with a rod or shown the barrel of a gun. Those who couldn't swim clung tightly to a rope that was suspended from our boat. These pirates were indeed cruel. They snickered, laughed at and taunted all of us.

Just before my mother's cousin jumped in the water, he quickly slipped a gold ring that he had been carrying in his pocket into his mouth. When the pirates spoke to him, he pretended to be mute, figuring this would ensure that he didn't lose what little he had left of his fortune. My mother's cousin soon realized that he couldn't keep treading water—he had to rest in order to survive. He approached the side of the boat, showed the pirates the ring in his mouth and offered it in exchange for reboarding the fishing vessel. Luckily, the pirates let him board, even though they could have just as easily taken the ring and left him to die out at sea anyway.

Unlike my mother's cousin, my father managed to bypass the experience of treading water in the open ocean. He was not a strong swimmer. So, in his brilliance, he believed he would stand a better chance of surviving if he played dead. It was not uncommon for people to die from starvation or heat exhaustion on these sea voyages, and so he lay limp on the floor amongst people's belongings. The pirates threw things on him, stepped on him and, when they did notice him, ripped his gold-framed glasses off his face.

My mother was wearing a tight-fitting jade bracelet. She knew the pirates would want it, so she quickly smashed the bracelet against the edge of the boat, shattering it into a few pieces. She did this out of fear, since she believed the pirates would chop off her hand to retrieve her jewellery. Just moments earlier, one of the pirates had brutally ripped an elderly woman's gold tooth out of her mouth.

We thought the horror would be over once the pirates had taken all our clothes, food and water, but it wasn't. They proceeded to take three young girls, crying and screaming, back to their boat. One of them was my eldest sister, who was fourteen years old.

My mother had heard horror stories of pirates sexually and physically abusing young girls, enslaving them in the sex trade indrustry. Now she feared they were going to do the same to her own daughter. My mother was quick to act. With five-year-old me in one hand and my four-year-old sister on her hip, she quickly and quietly told my eldest sister to stay calm, to obey the pirates and to always keep her eyes on us. Once back on their boat, the pirates made all three girls strip down before closely inspecting each of their bodies.

And then, just when we thought the pirates were about to sail away, and when my mother was sure she had lost a daughter, a miracle happened! Sirens began to blare and we saw a boat with red lights fast approaching us. The global community was aware of these brutal pirate attacks, which often included the raping of young women, even children, and the massacre of entire boatloads of people, violently clubbed or stabbed to death. The Thai government had refused to take any responsibility in preventing or punishing the perpetrators, and so, as a result, a few UN boats routinely patrolled these international waters. We all began screaming and yelling when we heard the sirens from afar. It had to be a UN boat coming to our rescue!

In the commotion, my mother madly cried out to my eldest sister: "Run and jump! Run! Jump!"

My sister, although scared, quickly did as she was told. She jumped over to our boat and wrapped her arms around my mother. In a mad panic, the pirates shoved the other two girls back onto our boat before quickly speeding off. They were obviously frightened of being caught. Although the UN boat did not actually approach us directly, their very presence in the area prevented the worst from happening to my family.

We were alive, but the pirates had taken our sources of light along with all our remaining food and water. In what was now a series of unfortunate events, our boat motor suddenly died, and we ended up floating on the open sea for four days. We couldn't steer and we couldn't propel ourselves. We were at the mercy of the ocean current. Many of us suffered heat stroke, and we had nothing but sea water to moisten our lips. Morale was very low; all we could do was pray. We knew we were close to Thailand when we could see local Thai fishing boats out for their daily catch. We cried out for help, but no one came to our rescue.

Fortunately, despite being sitting ducks, we encountered no more pirates. However, because we now had no light on our boat, we were invisible at night, and one night narrowly missed colliding with a big cargo ship. Grace—God's grace.

My brother's eyes lit up as he recounted this particular part of the story:

> I distinctly remember that night. It was shortly after our boat's engine had died. Everyone was asleep when I felt a sudden wave that literally lifted up our boat. I expected us to sink shortly after, believing we would be goners for sure. Then, from the corner of my eye, I saw two fins, one on either side of the boat. I had to rub my eyes to ensure I wasn't dreaming. There was a creature under us! It had to be a whale or large fish, or two. It was clearly taking us somewhere. It was a short ride and it seemed as if it had interceded to give us a 'push' toward land.

My brother tells me that I witnessed this event with him, but I was only five at the time and couldn't remember it. As my family began to awaken, my brother shared his story of the whale. Many of them just laughed at him and told him he had been dreaming. But shortly thereafter, our boat got stuck in a sand bar—we could now see land! While my brother insisted that a whale had saved us, everyone in the boat was in utter elation. Our nightmare of a boat ride was coming to an end.

The sand bar was about 500 metres from shore, so all at once, everyone decided to jump into the water and swim the remaining distance. In the frenzy, our boat flipped over from the quick displacement of weight. Many of us did not know how to swim. My father quickly found my grandma. My mother had my youngest sister in her arms. My aunt had me, and my mother's cousin had my third sister. The rest of my siblings fended for themselves. Our family quickly banded together and grabbed each other's hands. Our hands soon united with the hands of other members from our boat, forming a long human chain.

The ocean current was strong and was pulling us away from shore. The water was too deep for many of the women and children to stand, and so my brother, who had taken swimming lessons, began transporting individual family members to shore while my mother's cousin served as one of the anchors to the human chain, pulling people toward land. My aunt recalls being terrified. What kept her going was her will to survive and the sole thought of making it to shore.

There was light at the end of this tunnel. Although we were soaking wet, we had all survived. We were overjoyed and rejoiced in simply being alive. Our horrific ocean journey was over. When we looked back to our boat, all we saw was a shipwreck. Our boat had disintegrated before our eyes. It was a miracle that it stayed together as long as it had, remaining intact just long enough for us to reach Thailand.

We were quickly spotted by locals in the neighbouring village and were reported to government officials. We were now officially 'illegal refugees'. Protocol dictated that we were to sit and wait for the government officials to arrive.

When one family in the village realized that we were Chinese, even originating from the same village in China, Chaozhou, they cried out "Ga Gee Nung," which means "we are family." In China, it is common for families to offer extreme hospitality to strangers from the same village or with shared cultural roots. They gave us a bite to eat and water to drink, let us use their shower and even gave us dry clothes. My aunt remembered being so relieved and blessed to feel clean water on her filthy body and to have food to fill her empty stomach.

Due to the sheer volume of people leaving Vietnam by boat, the Thai government didn't have enough space to house us in the closest refugee camp, so we stayed in the village's crematorium with other refugee families for about two months. Meanwhile, my second aunt, who had stayed behind in Vietnam, was waiting anxiously to hear from us. We had told her that we would telegraph a message to her from Thailand after ten days of travel. As much as we wanted to contact her, that was the last thing on our minds. She went stir-crazy waiting to hear from us! She had intended to call the authorities if she didn't hear from us in one week's time, and she had already waited more than a month. We finally contacted her during the fifth week after our departure.

Although our story may seem unique, it is estimated that about two million people left Vietnam over the course of twenty years following the Vietnam War. Of those, about 800,000 arrived safely in another country by boat. It is believed that 200,000 to 400,000 Vietnamese died at sea due to pirate attacks, storms, starvation and poor conditions brought about by overcrowded boats. We were some of the fortunate ones whose boat ride had a happy ending.

My third aunt, whom we had hopes of finding once we reached Thailand, was one of the many who fled Vietnam by sea and were never seen again. We speculate that she was likely killed, beaten or captured during a pirate attack. It was reported that children saw their mothers beaten, raped or killed and that mothers watched their children sold into slavery or prostitution—even girls as young as six years old. Many never recovered mentally, and some ultimately committed suicide.

I recall reading an article that broke my heart. A father had witnessed his sixteen-year-old daughter being repeatedly raped by a crew of pirates. The ordeal was so violent that she hemorrhaged from the force. The violent assault against her body and spirit continued well after her body had given out. They had violated her over and over again before tossing her lifeless body overboard like a piece of garbage. Although her father's life was spared, he never recovered from the trauma and the loss. This is only one of so many haunting stories of the evil that was wrought on those seas. I am so grateful that this was not my sister's fate. I shudder to think what that ending would have meant for my family.

When I was younger, I frequently asked myself, "If God exists, why was this allowed to happen?" But as I have grown, I can say without a doubt that it was not God who was responsible for these heinous acts—we human beings were. Could God have stopped these acts from happening? Yes, but we are on Earth, not in Heaven. We are given free choice. This life is but a blip in the enormity of time. The pain and suffering we feel—and we will all endure some form of suffering, albeit to varying degrees—is a must in this lifetime. It is the question "Where do we go from here?" that truly matters.

4

Refugees in Thailand

With the life-threatening danger of pirates behind us, and with our feet firmly placed on dry land, we now faced a new obstacle—moving from Thailand to a Western or European country. It had always been our plan to move, we just never envisioned it unfolding in this way. After two months of living in the village's crematorium, the Thai government escorted us to a refugee camp called Lum Pi Ni, near Bangkok, where our family stayed together in one section of a small dwelling. There were no beds, but we recognized how fortunate we were to have made it thus far without much tragedy. We were hopeful that we would see my third aunt at the camp.

Once we settled into our new space, we began to evaluate our surroundings. As refugees, we were not allowed to cook our own food since the intent was that our stays would be short-term, lasting at most a few months. Instead, food was provided. All we needed to do was show up with a plate at a specific place and time, and meals would be provided from different embassies. Because we spoke both Vietnamese and Cambodian, we often previewed what each provider served before bringing food home.

Within a few months, we were moved to another camp, which consisted of an array of abandoned buildings. Although we now had beds, unlike at the previous camp, there were still no stoves or fridges. We ate what was provided to us. Later on, my aunt witnessed that the greens were not cleaned before cooking, and because vermin, like rats and insects, were running rampant, she suspected they too likely ended up in our meals. As a result, my aunt was determined to not to eat what the camp provided.

It was amazing to see that even in the camps, there was a clear socio-economic divide. While some people took on jobs to procure what money

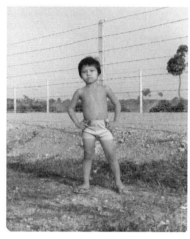

Five-year-old me at the camp

they could, others were 'living it up' on money that had been wired to them by family living elsewhere. My mother began working for a seamstress to earn extra money so we could eat cleaner food. Although we were not permitted to leave the camp, goods could be exchanged with Thai citizens through the chain-link fence.

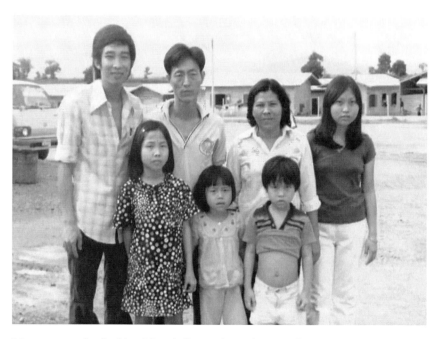

My parents, a family friend (top left), my three sisters and me; two siblings are missing from the photo

Because residents in this camp were only meant to live here short term, no school system was available for the children. Therefore, my eldest sister was able to go out daily to see what food was being offered free of charge and bring home whatever looked good. Whatever extra money we had was used to supplement our meals.

Every day, government officials from different countries set up stations to entice refugees to apply to immigrate to their country. Even before arriving at the camp, our family had hoped to seek asylum in Australia, France, Canada or the United States. We knew that these four countries were democratic nations, not currently involved in war, and a perfect place to raise a family. Australia was very selective about who they would admit. The United States was accepting refugees, but one would have to live on an 'American' island, Guam, for up to five years before setting foot on continental American soil. This was to give the US government time to figure out in which part of their country they wanted the new immigrants to settle.

My aunt desperately wanted to leave the camp, and she found out that Canada was not only openly accepting refugees but was also offering the quickest processing time. She was further enticed by rumours around the camp that even picking up garbage in Canada was a viable vocation. Because both my fourth aunt and my mother's cousin were single with no dependants, they would be granted quicker entry as compared to a family with children and seniors. Knowing these things, we collectively agreed that the easiest thing would be to all move to Canada.

When my aunt was screened by the Canadian government officials, they told her that because she was a young, single woman, it was best that another adult from our group go with her. Since my mother's cousin was also desperate to leave, they agreed to travel to Canada as a pair. Within five weeks, they were slated to restart their lives in Calgary, Alberta.

Both my aunt and my mother's cousin kept in touch with my family through long-distance telephone calls to the refugee camp while they started their lives in Calgary. The Canadian government covered the cost of their first month's rent and food, and a church was enlisted to help them get settled and to develop a sense of community. The government provided funds for them to learn English, and the church helped my mother's cousin find job opportunities.

He quickly found a job working at a restaurant and rented his own apartment, separate from my aunt. After my aunt's first few months in Calgary, she moved in with some of her new friends from church. It was important that my aunt could lean on the support of her church friends. Despite living with a roommate, it was still a lonely and scary place for a young, single immigrant woman. She saved all the money she made from working as a waitress. Although that didn't amount to very much, my aunt felt it was necessary to send money back to Thailand, to help us out in the camp. She anxiously awaited our arrival in Canada.

Unfortunately, our family's admittance process was delayed because both my father and my grandmother were suspected to have contracted tuberculosis. Luckily, the Canadian government was willing to cover any cost associated with their treatment, but they would need assurance that both of them were clear of any infectious disease before allowing them entry. It was during this waiting period that my father requested that we not be transferred to Calgary like my aunt and my mother's cousin. He wanted to settle in a warmer part of Canada.

Our camp was situated close to the water. At first, I was shocked to see boats drifting ashore with dead passengers, often men, since most pirates killed the men and spared the lives of the women and children. There seemed to always be a mass frenzy of people flocking to process and identify new refugees, hold funerals and cremate bodies. I soon settled into the routines of living at the camp, and this became the norm. Life was rather boring. I was now six years old, still mischievous, and there really was nothing for me to do all day.

One day, my brother was asked to watch over me while my mom was working and my father was at the local coffee shop. He was a young teenager who had no interest in babysitting. I decided to fly my kite, something I routinely did, except that on this particular day, I noticed that I could get more height if I flew it from the rooftop of a two-storey building, where there was more wind action.

On the roof, there was a staircase that led up to a smaller observation deck, which was about ten feet from the top of the roof and had no railings. Naturally, I wanted to be as high up as possible, so I ventured upward. I was so determined to get that kite to fly that I got lost in the moment and forgot where I was—I lost my footing. Because there was no railing and no caregiver to prevent me from falling, I fell ten feet from the observation deck onto the hard surface of the rooftop. As far as I knew, no one had any idea where I was. Luckily, a woman from the camp had seen me head toward the building with my kite and had heard me scream when I fell. She found me lying unconscious, with my kite nearby.

News of my fall spread like wildfire across the camp. My eldest sister was the first family member to get to the rooftop to identify me. Although there was no sign of blood, the woman who had found me instinctively knew I needed immediate medical attention. She was truly my angel. I was quickly taken to the camp's infirmary where I faded in and out of consciousness, and my head was swelling. My mom recalls wailing in the hallway outside the camp's infirmary—desperate for answers and for someone to help me. We didn't speak a word of Thai, as Thailand was always meant to be a brief stop on our journey. So now here she was, trying to communicate with the Thai nurse through a camp translator. In short, the nurse told my mother that I was in critical condition and that they had to find a way to remove the excess blood pooling in my cranial cavity. They feared that the blood would coagulate and form blood clots, preventing proper blood flow and thus permanently damaging parts of my brain.

I was suffering from head trauma due to a fractured skull. I needed a neurosurgeon to relieve pressure on my brain tissue to prevent death or severe disability. What were the chances of my survival? All odds were stacked against me. I was a six-year-old boy, not a celebrity or a child from a wealthy family or government official. For goodness' sake, I was in a refugee camp! But God stepped in. A neurosurgeon from the Western world, who happened to be a member of the Thai king's medical team, was vacationing nearby. God made sure this doctor heard my story and was so moved that he would go on to perform the first pediatric brain surgery of this magnitude in Thailand.

There were many inherent risks. There was a chance I could die, but the surgeon told my parents it was more likely I would enter a permanent vegetative state from which I would never awaken; become a quadra/paraplegic; or have a mental disability affecting my cognitive ability and/or social and emotional behaviours. My parents agreed to the surgery and did the only thing they knew how to do—they prayed.

When I awoke after the surgery, I did not recognize anyone; I was suffering from amnesia. I tried to scream, but no audible sound was heard. I cried and I was scared. I had a tube inserted into a secondary opening in my throat, had no control over any of my limbs, and I was in excruciating pain. My parents were horrified. The doctor mentioned that my erratic behaviour could become permanent.

The refugee camp allowed my mother to leave the camp to stay with me at the hospital while I recovered, but refugee camp officials expected her to travel back to the camp every few days. She would do laundry and update the family on my recovery.

My mother instinctively knew that what she was witnessing, what was happening to me, was beyond her control. She knew the only one who could help was not of this world. Because the Buddhist faith is strongly entrenched in Thai culture, there was a floor in the hospital dedicated for patients and their families to visit and pray. It was here that my mother became a devout Buddhist. She visited this floor at least once a day during my recovery period. She even refrained from eating meat, and both she and my father shaved their heads as an act of obedience and sacrifice.

Over the course of the next few weeks, my parents witnessed my memory slowly returning. My mother also suffered each time she saw me cry in pain whenever the nurses came to give me shots, move my limbs to prevent atrophy and when I attended physiotherapy to relearn how to use my arms and legs. In later years, my mother would show me the scars

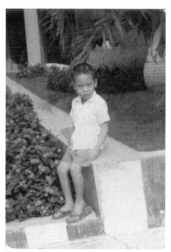 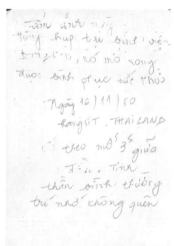

November 16, 1980: Photo taken after
I was discharged from the hospital in Rangsit, Thailand

where I dug my nails into her arms to share my pain with her because I had no voice to tell her what I was feeling.

Miraculously, I was discharged from the hospital after one month.

Later that year, in May 1981, the Cabinet of Thailand decided that two refugee camps for Vietnamese boat people, Songkhla and Laem Sing, would be closed and their seven thousand residents moved to Phanat Nikhom. Our whole family was yet again relocated to a new refugee camp, our fourth one. Then, about two months later, on July 6, 1981, we left for Vancouver, Canada.

5

Arriving in Canada

There has always been confusion around my birthdate and age. In the process of coming to Canada, my mother changed my age—reporting me as being one year younger—to ensure that I wouldn't have too difficult a time in school. But in the craziness of dealing with the paperwork to enter Canada, Mom also reported my birth month and date using the Julian calendar, stating that I was born December 24, 1974. Based on the Gregorian calendar, my actual birthdate is January 6, 1974.

I was born in the year of the Water Ox, which parallels many of my behaviours: I am quite direct, hardworking, persistent and loyal, but I am also stubborn, hate change and have a quick temper. After careful reflection by my wife, it is clear my mother's inaccurate reporting of my birthdate was predetermined—destined to be. Our paths never would have crossed if I had been put in the correct grade for my age, nor would my Julian calendar birthdate carry the significance of coinciding with Christmas Eve. (Did you know that there is no solid biblical evidence that Jesus was actually born on December 25? This date was first listed as Jesus's birthdate in a fourth-century Roman almanac—nearly four hundred years after his birth! Many speculate this date was chosen to coincide with the pagan winter solstice celebration.) It seems that Jesus and I both have inaccurate birthdates!

Like my aunt and my mother's cousin before us, the Canadian government sponsored us for our first year in Canada. This meant that our basic needs were covered. When we arrived in Vancouver, we stayed in a motel on Kingsway, near Boundary Road, for three weeks. From there, the government provided us with funds for a two-bedroom suite in South Vancouver.

Being refugees from a non-Anglophone nation, my parents did not speak English well, and by North American standards, we were considered a big family. Back in the refugee camp, my parents had heard rumours that one didn't need to worry about hardship in Canada: "Canada is so rich that even its streets are paved with gold!" Mostly, my parents were just grateful to leave the camp and to start a normal life. Both of them had to work to ensure we had food on the table and a roof over our heads. While all of us kids were in school during the day, my mother worked as a seamstress in a manufacturing company, and my father picked up odd jobs here and there, eventually finding work at a fish cannery. To make ends meet and to cover any extra expenditures, all able-bodied family members went berry picking during the summer months. Because my parents were often not home, my eldest sister was in charge of making dinner and managing the day-to-day chores around the house, while my brother earned extra cash as a dishwasher and paper boy. My brother, much like my father, was working long hours to financially assist the family.

Although my parents stayed together, it was clear that their arranged marriage was not based on love but rather on duty. My father was the typical Asian father: his job was to work and bring home money to run the household; my mother's was to cook, clean and manage all household matters (on top of her seamstress job); children were meant to be seen and not heard, and we were expected to respect our father and believe that he was always right.

Grandma Ngo, my father's mother, was an integral part of my life. She was consistently present, and she only spoke to us in Chauanese, the Chinese dialect from Chaozhou. Because of her, I was fluent in this dialect for ten years. As a youngster, I often had a hard time falling asleep, and I was obsessed with television, which meant that more often than not, I fell asleep while watching a show. Every night, my grandma would wake me up and tell me to go and sleep in my bed.

I was ten when she passed away from stomach cancer, at the age of seventy-six, toward the end of July 1984. After her passing, I would still, quite literally, hear Grandma Ngo waking me up, telling me to head to my room after I had fallen asleep on the couch. After a month of consistent encounters with my grandma, I finally told my mother what was happening and that I was scared. My mother then quickly prayed to our ancestors, telling my grandma that although we loved and missed her, she couldn't let us see her. Her job was done here, and she had to move on. I never saw Grandma Ngo again after that.

As our family became accustomed to living in Canada, we were able to focus on enjoying each other's company. We recognized the importance of taking care of each other, and truth be told, even though we were poor, I felt we were happy. Our family get-togethers were heartfelt—full of smiles and laughter. Because my eldest sister was my main caregiver, we developed a close relationship and had a very deep respect and love for one another. Being the first born, she had quite the load on her shoulders. She raised my youngest sister and me as if we were her very own children. She was often the first person I saw when I woke up and the last person I'd see before I went to sleep. She was there to both discipline us when we stepped out of line and to encourage us when we were down.

During these early years, I attended two elementary schools, Moberly and Weir. I was only at Moberly for a few months until my parents could afford a larger place for us to live. It was at George M. Weir Elementary School that I recall my life in Vancouver really beginning to take shape. When I started in grade two, I didn't speak a word of English, and even though I was technically older than my classmates, I was scrawny. But I was a quick learner who was motivated to fit in, and so I picked up English relatively quickly by watching a lot of cartoon television shows like *Transformers*, *He-Man*, *She-Ra* and *Super Friends*, and by playing with the neighbourhood kids. I easily made friends and was well-liked by my peers.

It was when I was partway through elementary school that my family and I all adopted Western names. It was my eldest sister who named me Wilson. When I asked her why she picked this name, she told me that she couldn't remember. It must have been something she had heard and liked the sound of.

I loved elementary school. I remember my first crush was on a girl in my class named Joanne. She was nice and pretty, and every boy in the class liked her too. I remember being so distracted by her beauty that I fell on my face. Unfortunately, the feeling wasn't mutual. Another vivid memory is of participating in the school play, *Dragon Tale*, in grade seven.

I played a knight and had a singing line, and although I was excited to have the part, I was going through puberty and remember being quite embarrassed that my voice cracked during the performance. I later found out that one of my classmate's parents had, of course, video-recorded this performance, so lucky for me, it lives on in posterity.

By 1986, both my eldest sister and brother had graduated from high school and entered the workforce. By this time, my parents had also begun the process of sponsoring our remaining family still left in Vietnam, my mother's two sisters, to come to Canada. To help my family financially, and to ensure that I had some spending money, I took over my brother's neighborhood paper route in the Killarney area in East Vancouver, delivering the *Vancouver Sun* and *The Province* newspapers by foot from a small red wagon. It was a rather labour-intensive job; I had to wake up early, and apart from delivering the papers, I frequently needed to knock on doors to collect payment. I recall stuffing newspapers into plastic bags with my mom and brother prior to deliveries on rainy or snowy days to ensure customers didn't get wet newspapers. And in the beginning, either my mother or brother tagged along to help me drag my full wagon and to make sure that I wasn't kidnapped or mugged. I held this job for about a year until my parents needed my help elsewhere.

Meanwhile, my father was nostalgic about his younger days back in Cambodia and dreamed of running his own business again. He didn't want to work long hours for someone else, so he invested in a laundromat in the Joyce-Collingwood area. In addition to providing laundering services, we also sold convenience items like cigarettes and snacks. Each of us had to take an afternoon, evening or weekend shift to relieve our parents. Even though we worked in pairs, we dreaded our shifts.

The laundromat business was short-lived. Besides our constant complaining about work shifts, the last straw came when my second sister, aged seventeen at the time, was assaulted by one of the patrons. There had been no one else in the laundromat that night, since my third sister couldn't work her scheduled shift. Years later, I asked my sister about her experience; here is what she told me:

> He was a young guy, in his early twenties. There was no one else in the laundromat. He appeared to be interested in purchasing some small convenience items. Then suddenly he pushed himself against me! I told him that my father was on his way back

to the shop and that he needed to stop. I then tried to grab the phone to call 911, but he had already ripped the wire connection to disconnect the phone line. My heart was racing. I told myself this couldn't be happening. I was not going to become a victim. I managed to get hold of a paring knife I had been using earlier to peel fruit. As I wielded this small knife, I kept repeating, over and over, that my father was on his way back to the store and would be here at any moment. Then suddenly, something scared him and he bolted out of the store.

In hindsight, God was gracious in that this young offender was a novice. He was shaking and hesitant during his attack, which likely caused him to withdraw and leave our shop. My sister quickly locked up the laundromat and called my parents. Shortly thereafter, my parents sold the business.

It was also around this time that my parents had saved enough money to purchase a house. Unfortunately, it was in Surrey, a suburb about thirty minutes from where we were currently renting. My family believed it would be wise for me and my younger sister to transfer out of Killarney Secondary School and attend the local neighbourhood high school, so we did. We lasted one week at the new high school before we hightailed it back to Killarney. We told our parents that we didn't feel safe attending the school in Surrey. While this new high school did have a reputation for being rather rough around the edges, in truth, I just really missed being around the friends I had grown up with.

By grade eight, I had formed a tight-knit group of friends. Admittedly, my group of friends did not have the best influence on me, and I would often skip out on math class to hang out with them. I was still trying to figure out who I was, and I soon found a passion for rugby and weightlifting. I developed a muscular physique from consistently working out and was proud of my newfound strength. It felt natural that I was often poised to fight, ready to show it off. To put it bluntly, my friends and I became bullies, picking on our classmates or riling up our opponents during a rugby game.

My family began to notice my obsession with strengthening my body, and my third sister became convinced that I was taking steroids. Soon I wasn't just poised to fight, I was fighting—even during band class, in the equipment room and after school, both on and off school grounds. To say the least, my reputation was not a positive one, especially in the eyes of our school principal. Even the girl I desperately wanted to impress wanted nothing to do with me.

By the end of grade nine, my grades were tanking, and my eldest sister was not impressed with me. She constantly lectured me and threatened to beat me if I didn't focus on improving my marks at school and stop physically hurting others.

As I entered grade ten, I decided it was time to make a change, but my so-called friends were not going to let me go so easily. Not only was I a source of entertainment, I was also a 'strong' member—a bulldog—in this teenage gang of hoodlums. To avoid them, I started hiding out in the library during breaks. I even became a library monitor and joined the Ecocentrics, an environment club. Suddenly, I found myself, a relatively 'badass' guy, hanging out with 'nerds'—the very same people I had once made fun of.

It was also around this time that I grew closer to Steve, who had joined my friend group the year before but whom I had immediately disliked—in fact, we had hated each other. But now, as I began to focus on school, Steve and I got closer, and he helped me to get my now ex-friends to back off and eventually leave me alone. It was also Steve who introduced me to Jesus. Reflecting on the night he invited me to join him at his church, Steve wrote:

> Wilson was family. He was my brother. He would charm my mom and my sister by telling them how good they looked. He would joke with my brother. On Sundays after church, I'd see his car parked outside my house waiting for me to get home. One night, I decided to invite him out to fellowship.

Prior to this, I had never given much thought to the existence of God, and my own parents were faithful Buddhists who practiced ancestral worship. I started going with Steve to church and joined him on his church retreats. I really enjoyed the fellowship. Steve literally "led me to the waters of Christ so that I could drink from His fountain." While I was attending this church, the congregants raised enough money to purchase land to build on a new site in Richmond. I recall physically digging and cleaning up the land on which the church would be built. The church, Cornerstone, still stands today on No. 5 Road in Richmond. Eventually, Steve stopped attending church regularly, but I continued to go for a little while longer.

Life became busier as I now had to spend more time studying and commuting via bus/SkyTrain to Vancouver for school every day. I also began forming a new circle of friends. I was becoming a geek, and I enjoyed it. There were now amazing teachers with whom I was able to connect, like Mr. Fukui (math) and Ms. Stager (English 11).

I'll never forget the day when I first tried to befriend a smarter peer. Looking back, it was quite comical. Here I was, a known bully, enrolled in a computer programming class. I purposely sat next to a smart, thin boy with spectacles who was literally shaking in his boots when I turned to ask him a question. We ended up becoming good friends.

My grades steadily improved. Inspired by Ms. Stager's class, I even started writing and publishing poetry.

Shadow

I know there's a shadow,
It keeps lurking outside.
Another lost shadow
That has no place to go.

I know of a dream
I could not conquer.
But to be conquered by this dream,
Breaking my heart into little pieces.

I know of a girl
I could love forever.
But I am afraid to confront her,
Knowing the result could be fatal.

For what does a shadow know
Except to wander off
Leaving behind a trail
Of brok
      en hea
         rts,
And shattered dreams.

I am just another shadow,
Waiting for the day,
The day I would be lost
Following a dream.
As I look toward the sun,
I'm blinded with memories of you.
All I can see is my dark shadow—
The shadow of loneliness.

Once long ago,
I saw the world—
The world that lay within your eyes.
I remember longing to see your smiling face,
For only then would the sun agree to shine and brighten up my world.

Oh, how can I be such a fool
To tell you about my love.
For after that I dare not look,
For a fool will always remain a fool.

— Wilson Ngo, 1992

Graduation was both sad and joyous. It was joyous in that this was the day my class and I had been anxiously awaiting for years. (It was also the day that my beloved brother, with whom my bond had strengthened as we became older, had promised to give me his sports car.) However, it also meant being separated from the very people I had grown to love. I wasn't going to UBC like many of my friends. Instead, my brother had encouraged me to get my post-secondary diploma at a trade school so that I could enter the workforce quickly and with practical skills. I would be going to BCIT. My brother had said that my endgame should be to be employed in as little time as possible, and because the technology industry was booming in the early 1990s, his advice made perfect sense.

6

Meeting the Love of my Life

Believe it or not, I met the love of my life in grade eight. As I was literally chasing another girl down the hallway on the second floor at lunch, I noticed a girl laughing and pointing at me as she sat with her friend in front of the lockers just outside an English classroom. Not only was she cute, but she was laughing at me. I paused just long enough to hear her friend yell out to me, "Your fly is undone!"

Yes, that's how we unofficially met. I was instantly intrigued. She was not in any of my classes, but I found out that her name was Rose and that she was in my best friend's English class. Rose had given her phone number to someone who wanted help with their English homework, and my friends and I managed to get a hold of it so we could 'crank call' her. Rose got very annoyed after the third call and put her mom on the phone, who promptly yelled at us. My friends soon lost interest and stopped bothering her, but I couldn't let it go. There was just something about her that I couldn't quite put my finger on. Even though Rose continued to hang up on me, I continued to call her every week or so. I just needed her to know who I was.

In grade nine, we finally had two classes together—band and French. I played the baritone and she played the clarinet. We didn't sit close to each other—in fact, we never even spoke. I didn't have a positive reputation, and at the time, I was still a bit of a bully. By grade ten, I had finally transitioned out of my bad-boy image. I stopped playing rugby and began to join clubs instead. I also knew without a doubt that Rose would not be a part of my future if I continued to act the way I did.

As my grades improved and I began to hang out with a different crowd, I got into the habit of calling Rose nearly every day. Since I had to wait around for my daily ride home, I would also often follow her home, from a distance, to kill time after school and to make sure she got home safely. At one point, I told Rose I was interested in going after one of her friends, and she willingly helped me. I even enjoyed listening to her talk about her then boyfriend or crush. Yes, I secretly wished it were me, but it was better to have her in my life as a friend than not at all.

In later years, Rose would confess that she and her friends used to walk home playing Would You Rather, a game in which the player had to choose between two usually equally undesirable options. The humour was in having to choose the best of the worst. One of the rounds would usually include, "Would you rather go to the prom with Wilson or...?" It turns out that both of them would pick the other option 99 percent of the time.

In my many attempts to court Rose, she would gently avoid the subject, telling me that we weren't right for each other. She would tell me things like I deserved someone smarter, nicer, kinder—a better catch. She would suggest some of her friends as options and offer to set me up. I would even write her letters to tell her how much she meant to me. I will never forget the one letter she wrote back to me. I was so excited when I saw the letter in the mail, but my heart soon sank once I read the opening line: "Dear Sir." I recall being so appalled, dumfounded even. Rose was putting her foot down, telling me to give up. We continued to be friends after that letter, but I soon started dating other people. And although I really wanted to be with her, I was mostly glad we were still friends.

After a year, and just before our high school graduation, Rose broke up with her boyfriend. This was likely one of the reasons why I managed to do better than her on the English 12 provincial exam. Writing was never one of my strengths. She was always the one who proofread and edited anything I wanted to be perfect. Rose tended to be good at many things, and now I had one up on her. Of course, I rubbed it in her face! And I continued to remind her of this fact whenever I had the chance.

In reflecting back on life, I would often tell Rose that I enjoyed high school. Given the opportunity, I would love to travel back in time to do it again. I fancied seeing the look on the face of Rose's younger self telling her that she would marry me! This was in stark contrast to Rose's thoughts about high school. She loathed high school. "Never," she said. "I have no interest in redoing any assignments or writing tests and papers. That would be one of my worst nightmares! I may have been a good student, but no thanks. I like where I am now." To which I would respond that she was a loser.

Shortly after Rose became single again at the end of grade twelve, I also broke up with my girlfriend. I didn't give my now ex a good reason why, just that I felt we weren't right for each other. I remember throwing out all the gifts she had given me in the short time we were together, one of which was a beautiful glass paperweight. Later that day, my mom took the paperweight out of the garbage and put it back in my room, thinking I had mistakenly tossed it. But I didn't want any reminders of my now ex; that chapter of my life was over. This is essentially how I am still—I don't believe in loose ends or in holding grudges. When a relationship ends, it's truly over—there is no going back.

After high school, Rose and I attended two different post-secondary institutions. I was at BCIT and she at UBC. But some things didn't change. I continued to call her at least once a day, late at night—sometimes even falling asleep as she recounted the details of her day.

While Rose was enjoying her time at UBC, I was miserable at BCIT. In fact, I hated my first year. At BCIT, my English professor put me in a tutorial class for ESL students to improve my writing skills. I was horrified! By the end of my first year, I had failed two courses, and my graduation from BCIT would be officially delayed. I remember calling Rose the day I found out, and I seized that opportunity to ask her out. To a certain extent, you might say I guilted her into a date. (Even Rose thought so, telling me a few years later that she had considered it a 'pity date' at the time.)

So nearly two years after her "Dear Sir" letter, we went out on our first date. And while we continued to date, Rose was planning to gently break off the relationship within a few months. She never anticipated falling head over heels in love with me. I overheard her tell her friends how we met and came to be a couple:

I never imagined myself with him. I just wanted to prove to him that we weren't right for each other. I just wanted to put that idea to rest and remain friends. But Wilson did everything he could to show me that he was worth it. He was right. Wilson truly enriched me—made me a better version of myself. But most importantly, he knew how to make me smile.

I was quite the sap, and at the time, I was obsessed with '80s music. I started assembling and organizing love song cassette tapes to express my love to Rose. Even then, I knew Rose was the woman I wanted to marry. To celebrate our first Christmas as a couple, I purchased a gold ring with a heart and tiny diamond. If we weren't still in school, and if I had actually had enough money to support us, I would have asked her to marry me right then and there.

It was also around this time that my aunt, who was a hairdresser, was diagnosed with stage four breast cancer. Despite chemotherapy, the cancer metastasized to her brain within a year. She passed away quite young, leaving behind a loving husband and three very young sons, including a set of twin boys. I remember feeling quite saddened by her ordeal. I saw her every few months for a haircut and witnessed the side effects of her treatment: extreme fatigue, weight loss and hair loss. I would never have dreamed that this would foreshadow my own life.

To celebrate our first year together, I saved up a month's pay from working part-time as a line cook for a Japanese fast-food chain to buy Rose a gold bracelet. It was a rather thick, yellow gold chain with several dangling heart charms. I told Rose that the hearts represented my love for her, just like in the ring I got her for Christmas. What a lovesick puppy I was!

While I firmly believe that Rose and I now have a wonderful relationship and marriage, it wasn't always easy. For example, I personally believe that men and women can't *really* be friends. I've seen time and again that sex always gets in the way. So when Rose and I started dating, I suggested that no solo meetings with a member of the opposite sex be a condition of our relationship. If such an occasion were to arise, like through school or work, we would let the other one know ahead of time. This was especially important to me because Rose was naive, and she was perhaps *too* friendly. And I was the typical overprotective boyfriend, driving her to and from study sessions because I thought it was important that I made my presence known. More importantly, I didn't want to give anyone else the opportunity to drive her home.

Rose hated this condition of our relationship, but she understood how important it was to me. She was adamant that this condition went both ways, meaning I had to also refrain from socializing with women outside of work and school hours. I had no issue with that since most of my friends and co-workers were men, and I spent my free time at home or with Rose anyway.

Much of what I learned about relationships was from those of my brother and eldest sister. In fact, when my eldest sister first started dating, my mother insisted that she take me and my youngest sister with her on all of her dates. We were literally the third and fourth wheels in her relationship with her new boyfriend at the time. Fast-forward a few years to my eldest sister finding and marrying her true love. We were sad to see her leave our home but extremely happy for her to start her new life as a married woman.

My sister and my brother would often share both the positives and negatives of being in a loving relationship with their partners. We would all laugh and cry together as they recounted their precious moments with us. Their relationships framed what I would eventually want from mine. At one point, my brother experienced a difficult low in his relationship that involved him being falsely arrested for domestic violence. I recall that, upon hearing this news, I went outside to pound the grass until my knuckles bled. If ever there was a time that I learned to loathe someone, it was from this incident. But over time, God showed me that I had no right to be judgmental. Matthew 7:1 says, "Judge not, that you be not judged. For with the judgment you pronounce you will be judged, and with the measure you use it will be measured to you."

I eventually learned how to willingly forgive and let bygones be bygones.

At the beginning of our relationship, I used to tell Rose how important it was for the man to love the woman more than she loved him. I felt this would ensure that the man had no 'cheating heart', since a man only has enough blood for either his brain or his penis, but not both! It was perfect, then, that I definitely felt more vested in our relationship than she did.

Although Rose was expressive and communicated often, I knew she really only shared her opinion when needed. She was a great listener. And though I felt that I was a pretty good listener too, I'll admit I did tune her out once in a while. As our relationship continued to grow, others who knew us well often commented that we acted like an old married couple. We were often on the same wavelength. We could lift each other up and at the same time, lovingly make fun of each other. Rose easily finished my thoughts and sentences. And while there were times when she crossed the line, over the years, she helped me learn how to express myself rather than blow up in a fit of rage.

Although I was a loyal friend, I had character flaws. I was stubborn and as impatient as an ox. Certain things caused my blood to boil, and I would lose control and enter into a fit of rage. I hated to be nagged at and lied to, and I definitely did not like being told what to do. I could not be beaten into submission, and when my anger set in, I could not be easily reasoned with. I recall being so upset one night that I punched a hole in the wall of my parents' home. Although I felt badly that I had damaged their home, I just couldn't contain my anger. I knew that I had to physically release that tension from my body.

Pride was my vice. I was a 'man's man', a typical Asian male. I grew up with the popular Chinese idiom: "A man is only to bleed, and not to shed a single tear." It became my mantra. Tears were a sign of weakness. I did not readily open up to people, instead remaining guarded and pessimistic. I was judgmental and slow to trust others.

Rose was the polar opposite. But she learned from me to be more careful about who she trusted. I felt she was 'book smart' but not very 'street smart' and that she was naive to think that most people had good intentions. She could be quite the optimist, which I saw often set her up for disappointment. But then again, her optimism was a good balance for my pessimism.

I loved Rose enough to die for her, but dating her wasn't easy. Because she was the eldest in her family, she had chores that had to be done and therefore restrictions on her schedule. In particular, she had to be home no later than four thirty every day, even on weekends, to help prep for dinner. Because I was likened to a 'dirty little secret', our dates were sold to her parents as study sessions.

When we first started dating in May 1994, Rose discouraged the idea of my meeting her family. I, on the other hand, immediately told my family about her, and my mom insisted that I invite her to my youngest aunt's wedding, where I paraded Rose around, showing her off to all my relatives. But after a year of sneaking around, I felt it was time that I met her parents and made myself Rose's official boyfriend. I wanted to be able to knock on her front door to pick her up, rather than meet up with her and drop her off at the library by her house.

I recall that day very well. I was very nervous—actually, I was scared shitless! Rose's parents spoke to me in Chinese, and I knew how important it was for me to respond back to them in their language. I did my best, using the Chinese I learned from watching Chinese movies and television growing up. Though the meeting was brief, it was well worth it. I was one step closer to marrying the love of my life.

Our personalities complemented each other well, and because we started dating at a relatively young age, Rose and I were lucky enough to watch each other mature. We learned to compromise and to give each other strength and support, or silence and space to grow, when needed. Over time, we morphed into each other's sounding board. We grounded each other. We knew how to come 'home' if we strayed too far. Rose often told our friends, "Wilson is not the same person I started dating back in May 1994. I sometimes have to do a double take and wonder who I am with."

My own friends saw a change in me after I began dating Rose. At our wedding, Steve gave the best man's speech, stating:

> Now, let me tell you how I know Wilson to be the man he is today. He was always quite the fighter. And it seems like after high school, he went and got himself a coach. And the name of the coach was Rose.
>
> As some years went by, I was quite impressed how they stayed together. I was pretty sure who wore the pants in the relationship. I always wondered how she dealt with his manhood, or how I call it…tough love. Funny how nine years go by and Wilson is no longer the fighter he was. I see the coaching from Rose. Wilson learned to beat others in another way, by having more heart and compassion.
>
> And throughout nine years, I've seen Wilson jump from car to different car. Whether Honda, Toyota or BMW, hatchback, sports car or four-by-four, one thing was always constant, and that was Rose. His love for cars has been surpassed by his love for Rose.
>
> Wilson, I've known you for quite some time now. You have a big tough heart. I am sure that I speak for others as well when I say that I feel safe having you as my friend. I know you will always be there. It's funny how by tradition, I have this title as 'best man' when clearly, I see you as being the best.

As with any couple, staying together required commitment and hard work. There were several calls to prayer in the rare moments when we were ready to call it quits, and the Lord intervened to ensure we fixed our eyes on His plan. As much as I loved Rose, she could be selfish and take me for granted, which made my blood boil. Equally, I could be quite stubborn, chauvinistic and unfair in my thinking. But we always owned up to our mistakes. After one of our disagreements, her apology included a poem, reminding me that she loved and respected me and that our relationship was worth fighting for.

> Love is about giving in…and not giving up.
> Love is positive, not negative.
> Love is always about one, and not two.
> How much do I love thee?
>> I cannot count the ways,
>> for my love runs deeper than that of the deepest ocean,
>> and soars higher than that of the heavens.
> I can only ask for forgiveness and for your love…
>> for those are the things that are most precious.
> What good is half of a pair without the other,
>> as is me without you…

> — *Rose*

7

Living My Life, My Way

In my twenties, religion wasn't really an important part of my life. Though I had nothing against it, I wasn't going to go out of my way to become 'enlightened'. I wanted what any typical young man desired—a high-paying job, a new car, a nice place to live and a loving wife and children.

Rose described me as a loyal, sensitive and passionate man who worked hard and who stood behind and fought for what he believed in. She would often tell me, "You ain't no bystander! That's one of the qualities I love about you. I know that you will always protect me, but you really have to get your temper under control." Admittedly, I had anger management issues. So much so that I even scared myself sometimes. Looking back, I am rather ashamed of my actions and recognize I was very much a part of the problem.

In one such incident, I was at a local movie theatre with my cousin to enjoy a movie that I had been excited to see for some time. In the seats behind us were two younger guys who would not stop talking. I had given them several 'nice' reminders to please be quiet, to stop kicking the back of my seat, to please, if they wanted to talk, take their conversation outside of the theatre so that the rest of us could enjoy the movie.

They ignored me. Not only did they refuse to be quiet, but they had the audacity to talk back and swear at me. I told them that I paid good money to appreciate the movie without background noise, and after the movie, I told them in no uncertain terms that they were rude. In response, they threatened to beat me up. It was clear that one of them felt rather cocky about his strength and muscular physique. And me? I actually *welcomed* the opportunity.

We met up in the back lot of the mall, and before words could even be exchanged, my cousin jumped one of them. And though my opponent was rather strong, I was no weakling, nor a stranger to fights. At one point, I remember saying to myself, "Why won't this guy go down? I'm giving him all I have." Both my cousin and I only left the scene when our opponents had no strength to fight back.

I felt badly afterward and knew that I should have called an ambulance. In my anger, I couldn't think beyond my own rage. I hoped that his friend would take care of him.

As with every fight, I was left with a heavy-laden heart, which resulted in my calling Rose to confess my regrettable actions. She was always disappointed, and this time was no different. She wisely asked, "Why didn't you just tell the security guard or the movie attendants? They would have had the boys removed from the theatre or at the very least moved them away from you."

Rose was logical, but I also felt that she was judging me, and I longed for her approval. I was an impulsive man, and honestly, I wanted to appear strong, not weak. But now I see this was only an excuse. A part of me wanted to feel again what I had felt as a young kid, when I could (and did) easily 'dominate' another human being. After speaking with Rose, I was reminded that I was supposed to be a mature adult who knew better.

I pictured myself in my opponent's shoes. First, I thought about his mother. And then I remembered my own mother, sitting and crying over my bedside in Thailand after my fall. It pained me to think that I wasn't just physically injuring another person, but I was also hurting someone else's mother.

I strongly believe my episodes of explosive anger were a direct result of my oversensitivity and passion. And although Rose and I occasionally exchanged angry words during heated arguments, I never lifted a finger to harm her physically. In fact, I was often the one who was the first to apologize after a disagreement. It was important to me that we minimized misunderstandings and feelings of resentment as quickly as possible. This was in stark contrast to Rose, who, if it were up to her, would walk away and return to the issue the next day. She felt the need for space to clear her mind, formulate a solution and analyze the issue without input from others. For Rose, it was necessary that her thoughts were not influenced by others, mainly me.

In truth, her 'thinking' always scared me. Deep down, I was nervous she would second-guess our relationship. I didn't want her to leave me because of my anger management issues. My solution? I made it a point to be around when she was processing her thoughts. I would literally not leave her side until I felt confident that we were okay.

Provocations, giving me an excuse to allow my anger to rule me, seemed to follow me. And although I wasn't actively seeking a fight, it seemed like a dark cloud was always looming over me—even as I drove Rose home from her sister's graduation ceremony. While changing lanes, I accidentally cut off another car. I did the classic "I'm sorry" wave through my rear-view mirror and out my window. But the young driver in the other car was so upset that he decided to cut me off at the next intersection. Not only that, but he got out of his car at the red light and threateningly circled my car—in the middle of traffic in broad daylight! He probably thought I was a small guy and wanted to prove to his buddies how tough he was. That made my blood boil. I got out of my car, despite Rose's repeated pleading to "just ignore the punk kid." She yelled, "Wilson, you are better than this!"

But I couldn't stop myself. No—actually, a part of me didn't want to stop. Once the 'punk kid' realized I wasn't backing down, and once he saw that I was physically stronger than he was, he decided to remove his belt and call to his friends for reinforcement. In my head, I'm wondering, "What? Did he think he was going to beat me with his belt? Really? He needed his friends to back him up too?"

The traffic light had by now turned green, and we were stopping traffic. I ended up getting back in my car, not only because of Rose's insistent stare, but also because cars behind us had started honking. The punk kid and his friends also got back into his car but continued to tail me, egging me on.

Because I had Rose in the car, I decided to do the 'right' thing. I was going to drop her off at home, since she only lived a few blocks away, and then I was going to find this punk kid to give him a piece of my mind! Rose was clearly not happy with my irrational decision. She told me that if I went after that car, our relationship would be over.

But I was too hotheaded. I couldn't control nor contain this feeling inside me. At this point, I didn't care what Rose said. Once she exited my car and shut the door, I drove off in pursuit. After five minutes of driving around the neighborhood, I finally cooled off. Once I was able to think rationally, I went back to Rose's house. Her mom told me she wasn't home.

This was not a good sign. I knew that Rose must have gone out for one of her 'thinking' walks, which meant she couldn't have gone far. I could still rectify the situation. When I finally found her fifteen minutes later, she said, "I'm done, Wilson. It's over. I can't be with someone who has such an explosive temper. I know you love me, but your anger scares me."

That hit home. I wasn't about to let her go, especially over some punk kid. I did what any guy so head over heels in love would do—I apologized. I told her how sorry I was and that I understood my temper was a problem. I told her that I would never hurt her. Lucky for me, she stuck by my side as I worked on dampening and controlling my hot temper.

There were at least two more physical altercations that happened before I finally put my fists away. One happened just as I had finished my evening ski run on one of our local mountains. I used the washroom and decided to change out of my ski wear in the stall. Within minutes, a drunk guy was pounding on the stall door telling me to hurry up. I told him that I would be out in few minutes. The drunken skier continued to yell, insisting that I had to get out of the stall immediately because he had to "take a shit." I was getting agitated and reminded him there was another washroom stall, but he continued to pound on the door. When I came out of the stall, the drunkard began to swear at me and even moved to throw a punch. I couldn't resist; I knocked the guy out. Security was notified, but in the end, no charges were laid.

After the incident, I called Rose and drove directly to her house. When she opened the door, she had this look that read, "What were you thinking?" When she noticed the blood stains on my shirt, her expression changed from disappointment to concern. "Oh my God! Are you okay? There's blood on your shirt!" I laughed and said, "It's not mine."

Rose's parents came downstairs shortly afterwards, asking about the blood on my shirt. I explained that I had been in a fight and that the blood wasn't mine. On a normal day, Rose's mom was hard to impress, so you can imagine that on this day, she was quite upset. She kicked me out of their house! I knew she felt I wasn't good enough for her daughter. And she was probably right. In retrospect, it all seems quite comical. I recall the drunken skier telling the security guard that he didn't mean to cause all this trouble, he had just wanted to use the washroom.

It would be the next incident, however, that would finally cause me to reconsider using my fists to solve any of my problems. I used to work part-time at a Japanese fast-food teppanyaki joint in one of the local malls. On this particular day, I was working the closing shift with another employee. He was about ten years older than me, in his early thirties with a young family. I can't remember what we were arguing about in the back room after closing, but he said something that provoked me. I warned him to stop, but he didn't. And when he wouldn't, I punched him, knocking him to floor and giving him a black eye. Although I knew this was not acceptable conduct in a work environment, I couldn't control myself, and as always, my rage took over.

Upon hearing what happened, my boss called me the next day to fire me. But because I had already made plans to quit, I really didn't care. What sparked me to change was, in fact, my usual after-fight discussion with Rose. I started picturing myself as the guy I had injured. What did he say to his wife and family when they saw his black eye? I likely hurt him enough that he would have to take a few days off work—meaning loss of income and less money for their family. How would his children feel, seeing their dad injured and unable to work? I reflected on the fact that I was the one who had caused this pain.

I always believed that I had enough sense to never hurt my family, that I would always have control with the ones I loved. But soon God would test me.

Being so close in age to my youngest sister resulted in a lot of friction between us growing up. We were constantly at each other's throats. I used to play stupid pranks on her, one time even breaking open a beehive without telling her, just so that she would get stung. Yes, I was rather evil. Although I loved my sister, I disliked her strong feminist perspective and her need to always be right. (Of course, I now know that I, too, had a hard time accepting being wrong.) But more so, I hated people rubbing my embarrassments or failures in my face.

My youngest sister and I both lived in my parents' home as we attended post-secondary institutions. The next natural milestone for me was to move out. However, I was comfortable being fed and not really having to pay rent. I saw this as savings—more spending money for me. One day, my younger sister and I got into a fight while my parents were away on vacation—a heated argument over the TV remote. There was only one TV, and we each wanted to watch our shows. I was not willing to compromise, and neither was she. My sister told me that I was not the "king of the house" and definitely not the boss of her.

I lost control. The feelings of rage and anger took over. I told her to back off, but when she didn't, I threatened to beat her. That's when she pulled out a kitchen knife to defend herself. Luckily, one of my other sisters was home and able to stop us from hurting each other. We were both so out of control that our sister picked up the phone to call the police. When I left the house to cool down, I called Rose. It was time to move out.

In retrospect, moving out was what I needed to truly grow up. It was only after moving out that I learned more about myself and began to financially plan for my life.

I grew up without many material comforts. I had no silver spoon, and I honestly believe that growing up relatively poor was a big part of God's plan for me. It is only in our hardships that we grow to appreciate what we have. Until I started working, much of what I had were hand-me-downs or gifts from my eldest sister. Throughout most of high school, I picked up odd jobs here and there to make extra money for bus fare, food and clothing. My eldest sister even got me a job as a dishwasher at a Mexican restaurant in Kitsilano before I was legally allowed to work. When I did reach the legal working age, I became a line cook at the food courts in Oakridge Mall and Surrey Place Mall. Shortly thereafter, I worked at a watch repair shop, replacing watch batteries for customers.

Like most young adults, I had materialistic desires. I was crazy for cars! My first car was a new, basic model, 1995 green Honda Civic hatchback. My mom paid for my first year of car insurance, and I borrowed $2,000 from my younger sister to use as a down payment. The feeling of owning my own car was unbeatable. Thus began my insatiable desire to constantly have a new car. Over the course of the next five years, I owned six different vehicles!

With all these cars, you would think I was going through a mid-life crisis. Because many of my first few cars were Hondas, the Honda car dealerships and financing departments really liked me. My family kept telling me that I was throwing my hard-earned money down the drain. They were right. I was paying too much in interest and losing money from depreciation. I also didn't have a business at the time to write off any of these expenses. But I didn't care what anyone thought, because it was *my* money that I was spending, and I was happy.

Although I always had an eye for nice things, my extravagant indulgences didn't really begin until I started working for a medical imaging company, about seven years after I graduated from BCIT. It was with this job that I could finally afford to pay for our wedding. I believed that by being married, I would have a fresh start to build a new life with someone. So, after four years of dating, followed by a lengthy five-year engagement, Rose and I 'tied the knot' in the summer of 2003.

At our wedding in Vancouver, Rose presented a speech in front of our 270 guests. She spoke of how we didn't get to choose our families—God did—and that no matter how badly we felt about any situation, there was always a reason and a purpose for everything. I think it is human nature to want what you don't have, and I wanted to create my perfect family—starting with being the perfect husband and father, something I felt was missing when I was growing up. But I recognized that although I strongly wished for a father who met my needs, my father had shaped me to be the person I was.

That, too, was a part of God's plan. I am loyal and faithful because I witnessed first-hand what happened to the ones I loved when a marriage wasn't knit together with true love and honesty. I saw how selfish actions hurt a spouse, and for that reason, I knew I had to be open to compromise. It was in these moments of reflection that I learned how to become a good son, brother and husband.

Shortly after our wedding, I was itching to buy another new car. This time, I wanted to buy a luxury SUV for Rose. I wanted her to be safe, but secretly, I also didn't want to feel guilty about splurging on things for myself. It took a lot of convincing; I had to build a case for my expensive purchase. Thankfully, this didn't prove too difficult. Since my job required me to be out of town for at least 60 percent of the year, and I planned to work from home on the days I was in town, we wouldn't need to have two vehicles. I told Rose that we could trade in both our current ones for a nicer one, for which she would be the principal driver. I promised to take the bus or ride my electric scooter for at least a year to make up for this new expense.

Rose was skeptical of my commitment to take public transit or my scooter, but I did fulfill my promise. While many of my colleagues at work laughed and joked about my 'ride', many more of them were quite impressed with my commitment to Rose. Sure enough, this positive experience also led to my own indulgences in luxury cars for years to come.

My love of cars was inherent in me as a young boy, and my love of driving began before I could legally step on a gas pedal. Consequently, I ensured that Rose and I took a few long road trips every year—either down south to the United States or east to Calgary and Banff. (I was not a speedster, except for one speeding ticket in Golden, BC, en route home from Calgary—acquired despite my use of a radar detector.)

I took every opportunity I could to have my employer approve a road trip over a flight for anything that required my working out of town. My most memorable trip was driving from Vancouver to San Jose, California. I recall driving in my convertible with the top down, '80s music blaring, wearing my sunglasses and baseball cap. Since I was alone, I sported my infamous white Calvin Klein tank top, which my friends jokingly and somewhat offensively referred to as a 'wifebeater'.

Because I enjoyed the cool breeze on my face and blowing through my hair, I completely forgot about how damaging the sun was. By the time I arrived at the hotel after a full day of unprotected sun exposure, I looked like a raccoon! I did my best to avoid removing my sunglasses in public; however, I did have to show my full unobstructed face when I met the medical team at the job site. In a way, my appearance broke the ice, as it allowed everyone to have a good chuckle.

With the exception of owning different cars, I wasn't into trying new things. When I found something I liked, I tended to stick with it. I often thought of this as loyalty. At least that was the excuse I'd tell Rose whenever she asked me to step outside of my comfort zone when it came to what I wore or what I ate. I did have a passion for accessories, so much so that some friends called me the 'metro man'. I always sported a nice watch and my wedding ring.

I was also conscious of my physique, though I loved to eat! Rose would frequently tell me that I had problems with self-control, as I would often overindulge. "Bingeing" or "binge eating" is what she would call it. She was right. Rose was often the one who had to put a stop to my indulgences or set a limit for me. And while I would give her a hard time about it, I knew that she was setting these boundaries because she loved me. Little did I know that the need for these parameter-setting measures was foreshadowing a future of health issues.

Shortly after we were married, my work consumed my life. As mentioned, I was working for a medical imaging company that required me to travel a lot. One particular year, I was away just over two hundred days! There were times when I literally came home to do a few loads of laundry and kiss my wife and the dog before flying out again. This obviously complicated our marriage on many fronts.

Although I was away from the person I loved most, I also made many new friends and developed positive relationships with doctors. One such relationship was with a doctor in Corpus Christi, Texas. He was so caring that when he was in town for product training, he came to Rose's lab appointment to review an ultrasound of a cyst in her breast. Another time, he pulled some strings so that I could get a complimentary CT scan at his hospital in Corpus Christi when I was there to perform a system upgrade. This scan revealed that I had degenerative bones in my spine due to my fall at the refugee camp in Thailand and that I had remnants of metal shavings in my brain from the resulting surgery.

As I entered my mid-thirties, more health issues began to pop up, including chronic kidney stones that would form every twelve to twenty-four months. My steady weight gain also led to an increase in blood pressure and cholesterol, and at one point, I was even borderline diabetic. My family doctor told me I had to lose some weight or start taking medication to alleviate the pressure on my organs. But I was defiant; I honestly believed I was untouchable.

At this point in my life, I chose to enjoy luxuries, like food and wine, without any care for my physical body. I was no longer treating my body like the 'temple' that it was—God's temple. I remember Rose telling me that we could go on a diet together. I flat out told her "No." In fact, eventually I altogether refused to eat things she made that I didn't care for. I would later come to regret this decision.

8

My Struggle with Faith

Although Jesus was a part of my life in high school, the importance of religion had petered off by the time I graduated. I was consumed by my desire to court Rose, earn spending money and finish my education. As things were checked off my life's to-do list, Christ did eventually come back into view.

Although I may not have been paying attention, God had still provided me with humbling experiences. On at least two separate occasions, I witnessed people nearly die in front of me. In both instances, I was compelled to provide them comfort and aid in what could have been their last moments of life.

One such time involved a young dad who was changing his car's flat tire on the side of the road. An oncoming vehicle lost control and hit his parked car, pinning him underneath his vehicle. His young child was confused and crying from the shock of the accident whilst restrained in the car seat. I saw it all unfold before my eyes and quickly called 911. The paramedics asked if anyone had anything warm to provide the man after finally prying him out from underneath his car. I offered my sweater without a second thought—the one that Rose had just gifted me.

Another time, about a year later, I witnessed a man have a heart attack a few metres in front of me as I was walking between job sites downtown. Once again, when the paramedics asked for a warm article of clothing, I offered my scarf, lovingly hand-knit by Rose.

In both instances, I went home in shock. These moments reminded me how fragile and precious life was. It made me re-evaluate the importance of family and my desire to not only live my life joyously, but also in a way that honoured the opportunity to live in community with others.

Although these tragedies forced me to think about death and the meaning of life, it was actually Rose's struggle to pursue God that sparked me to wonder more about Him too.

It was obvious to me from the beginning that Rose was spiritual. This was one of the things that first attracted me to her. Neither of us came from Christian families, but shortly after we began dating, she felt a void that needed to be filled and a prompting from the Holy Spirit to find a place of worship. Rose asked me if I would join her in her quest, and because it was so early in our relationship, I felt obligated to agree; however, since I had fallen off the faith bandwagon and was open to reconnecting with God, this request was palatable. Besides, this meant spending more time with Rose.

Up until this point, Rose had only been to a few Roman Catholic Sunday services and a few fellowship meetings at a local gospel hall. I, myself, had only ever been to a conservative Chinese Baptist church. We longed for a church of our very own to call home—one where we would genuinely feel like we belonged. Rose made a list of churches by thumbing through the Yellow Pages, carefully picking from different denominations among the ones that were relatively close to her home.

One of the first churches we visited together was a Pentecostal church in East Vancouver. We immediately felt the warmth that exuded from the congregation, and Rose was moved to tears during worship by the strong presence of the Holy Spirit. I could tell that Rose believed we had hit the jackpot. However, our perception changed as we transitioned out of worship and into a special healing service. Because we didn't understand the true power of the Lord, we were in a state of shock and disbelief at what we witnessed during the remainder of the service. How could people be falling to the ground once touched by the preacher? Why were people screaming and dancing? How could this be real? Why did we feel like we were watching something fabricated on TV? We left with more questions than answers and, to a certain extent, disappointed.

We were disappointed because we no longer felt this church was a good fit for us. In actuality, it was us who weren't yet a good fit for the church—we were the ones who weren't ready to accept what we had seen. We didn't have the foundation of faith necessary for us to believe in what we couldn't easily explain.

In our spiritual immaturity, I suggested we take a short break from church hunting. Rose was reluctant to stop, but she valued my opinion and saw the logic in taking a step back. During this break, she learned about an Alpha course being offered at a church in New Westminster. Rose had just received her driver's licence and didn't drive often, perhaps once or twice a month. She heard the advertisement on the radio while she was driving, and since there was no way she was able to remember the contact information after hearing it only once, she told God that she would attend if she heard about it again on the radio.

Sure enough, early one morning about a month later, Rose heard the same advertisement on the radio in her bedroom and immediately called the Lutheran Church in New Westminster. It would be a twenty-minute drive to attend this Wednesday evening class, and Rose was clearly committed to attending the full three-month course. Being her other half, I joined her. At this time, I had just started my job as an implementation specialist at a medical imaging company. About one month into the Alpha course, the company expected me to start flying out to job sites. This left Rose to attend the sessions on her own.

About two months into the program, the pastor running the Alpha course moved to another church and it was terminated. Because Rose had experienced spiritual growth and wanted to finish the course, she looked for other churches offering the series. Once again, I couldn't commit to the sessions due to work obligations, and Rose did not have a vehicle; therefore, she looked for a church along a bus route. This led her to Chinese Presbyterian Church (CPC) by Oakridge Mall in Vancouver.

In retrospect, I can now say that God truly works in amazing ways, as I see how these experiences were a part of His master plan for us. God didn't give up on us when we weren't ready to see His power. He waited for us. As long as we are open and willing to hear His voice, God will be there, in the background, ready to fill us with His grace.

CPC took the two of us on a great spiritual journey. The congregation was warm and welcoming, and alarmingly familiar. I remember telling Rose that several individuals reminded me of people from our high school. In hindsight, this was one of God's markers, encouraging us to stay rooted here for a while.

At this point, Rose and I were now officially engaged to be married. I recall the moment I looked at her and knew that I wanted her to be a part of my 'forever' life. As I mentioned earlier, if money hadn't been an issue, I would have proposed after dating her for six months. It took me four years to finish school, get a job and save up for a ring. I presented her with the ring a few months before she graduated with her first bachelor's degree. Although Rose had agreed to marry me, a part of me felt she wasn't 'all in'.

Together we decided on a long engagement, as she was pursuing another degree and didn't want to get married until she finished her schooling. I must admit that I wanted Rose to wear her engagement ring for selfish reasons, not only because we needed time to save money for the wedding, but more importantly, I wanted other men to recognize she was not available.

Our engagement ended up being five years long, and this too was planned by God. It was in this time that the both of us grew closer to not only each other, but also to Him. This was one of the missing pieces that Rose was waiting for—she wanted to marry a God-loving man.

We attended a marriage conference called Weekend Away in Kelowna in March 2003, where I recommitted my life to Christ. Rose told me that she had been praying for me for the last few years to entrust my life to God, as she had already done. Her faith in God was clearly deeper than mine, and she seemed more willing to give control of her life to Him. I believe this is why God gave her a vision. About a year before the conference, she felt God tell her that an older man in our midst would be the one to lead me to Him. When Rose told me this story, she giggled as she recalled wondering who that person would be and when it would happen. She kept thinking it would be an elder from our church, but it wasn't.

As God promised, it was an older gentleman—one of the presenters at the marriage conference. I was instantly drawn to him and his message on the importance of staying married and staying in love. He shared his struggle to make compromises and to overcome his own selfish desires in order to ensure his partner felt loved. He emphasised that the success of his marriage was rooted in the fact that God was at the core of their relationship. I could see how happy he and his wife were, even after many years, and I wanted that kind of a marriage for me and Rose.

I began to see it as my duty to be a God-fearing and loving husband. In this moment, I was also able to recount and see how God was present at every turn in my life. I was overcome with the Spirit and felt so blessed that God had gifted me with a life partner who made me want to be a better person. At the end of his presentation, the older gentleman asked anyone who felt moved by the Spirit to sign a commitment statement in our conference booklet. I felt compelled to sign my name, agreeing to follow and surrender my life once again to Christ, recognizing that He died so that I would be free of my sins and that He loved me unconditionally.

As I signed the booklet, I noticed Rose's eyes had welled up with tears. She had been quietly watching me. They were "joyful tears," she later told me, a confirmation from God that we were doing the right thing. I knew at that moment that drawing closer to God would also draw me closer to Rose.

We left the conference renewed. Rose felt complete, knowing that we were going to be married, our hearts knit together with God at the centre. God would always be with us, directing and reminding us how to treat, respect, listen to and love each other. We were to remember that when overtaken by selfish desires or anger during disagreements, we could turn to God to ask for wisdom, grace and help. The Bible verse from 1 Corinthians 13:4–7 (NIV) became a mantra for our marriage:

> [4] Love is patient, love is kind. It does not envy, it does not boast, it is not proud. [5] It does not dishonor others, it is not self-seeking, it is not easily angered, it keeps no record of wrongs. [6] Love does not delight in evil but rejoices with the truth. [7] It always protects, always trusts, always hopes, always perseveres.

If God weren't the focal point in our marriage, we would have had to put our ultimate faith in each other. In a perfect world, this would seem to make sense—it would mean loving each other and always putting each other's needs first. But this is an unrealistic expectation for anyone, as we are by no means perfect. I, for sure, am not perfect, nor will I ever be. I am riddled with flaws. Having God as our foundation and centre meant that I had someone to answer to. I wouldn't need to focus on adhering to, guessing or challenging expectations put on me. Instead, I could count on my relationship with God to mould me to naturally be a better and more caring spouse, as stated in Ephesians 5:25–27 (ESV).

[25] Husbands, love your wives, as Christ loved the church and gave himself up for her, [26] that he might sanctify her, having cleansed her by the washing of water with the word, [27] so that he might present the church to himself in splendor, without spot or wrinkle or any such thing, that she might be holy and without blemish.

Hence my love for God would keep me accountable to Rose. We were married three months later, on Saturday, June 28, 2003. We chose two songs to be sung at our ceremony: "The Power of Your Love" and "Be Thou My Vision." Both of these songs reference God as the source of our love and strength—a reminder to us that He is always watching, ready to catch us when we fall.

While the vows of our wedding and our commitment to each other were done in God's name, we also adhered to many of the traditional rituals of a Chinese wedding. One consisted of me picking up my bride from her mother's house before the wedding. This action serves as a symbol of the bridal family losing a daughter, like an official hand-off, the bride leaving one family to be received by another.

In Chinese weddings, it is also customary for the bridesmaids to pull pranks, also called 'door games', on the groom, to test his desire to marry his bride and to win approval from her family. I recall having to drink a nasty concoction that included hot sauce, vinegar, pop and other questionable ingredients that have remained unnamed. In yet another prank, one of my groomsmen dressed up as Rose, and I had to carry him around as part of a piggyback contest. Finally, before my bride could be 'surrendered' to me by her bridesmaids, I had to hand over a red packet containing money for them to share.

Although I had a blast, I was glad when the games were done so I could get on with our wedding festivities, which included me finding Rose and carrying her out to the living room filled with close friends and family from the bride's side for our first tea ceremony. This tea ceremony allowed Rose and me, the bride and groom, to express our gratitude, respect and appreciation to Rose's parents, officially honouring and thanking them for raising and supporting her. Rose's parents were using their finest China tea set. I recall feeling so happy kneeling in front of my new in-laws. I knew that upon passing the teacup to Rose's parents, not only would I be officially a part of her family, but she would also be a part of mine. After sipping the tea from us, Rose's parents said a blessing over us and handed us a red packet of money.

After a few photos at the bride's home, we drove about forty minutes to my parents' place for our second tea ceremony. Because I have a larger family, we served tea not only to my parents, but also to my married aunts and uncles, brother and sister. In exchange for each sip of tea, we were given red packets of money or jewellery.

To follow was our church ceremony. This was the part that would be most important and meaningful to me. Although I had been anticipating this day for a while, I was jittery and had spent most of the night before memorizing my vows to Rose.

Time passes and days go by.
With each sunset my love for you deepens,
and with each passing second I am left breathless,
to ponder how I would be without you.

It is these words that have bought me here today.
My life is incomplete unless you are a part of it.
You are my guiding light, and without you
I am hopelessly lost.

As I reflect back on my life, I realize that I have been blessed by the Lord because he has sent an angel to watch over me.
The Lord sent you to watch over me to help me through my struggles and celebrate my triumphs.

First we were strangers,
then we met, but we weren't too fond of each other.
Then we became friends,
and then we fell in love.
But this is just the beginning of our story.

The ceremony was followed by photos at Queen Elizabeth Park, a rest break and a lavish eight-course Chinese banquet. During dinner, I ended my speech by singing a song to my wife. The opening line to the song, "One Good Woman" by Peter Cetera, expressed exactly how I felt. I was so in love with Rose, and I just could not deny it.

Although I was elated to be officially married, I didn't feel like things had really changed. I was with the woman of my dreams, and now I had an extra dad, mom and sister. It wasn't until I visited my father-in-law the next day that I realized my wedding had altered his perception of life. Rose's dad was smiling when he greeted us at the door, but then after a few minutes, his eyes filled with tears. He explained that he felt like he had lost a daughter, even though she was standing right in front of him. Rose quickly told her father that his thinking was skewed. She tried to make him see the glass as half full and not half empty. "You didn't lose me! You gained a whole new family, Dad! You gained a son and his entire family, including his siblings!"

Upon hearing those words, Rose's father smiled and nodded. I only grew to love and respect him even more after that.

In an effort to save money, Rose and I decided to postpone our honeymoon in Hawaii to November, when ticket prices were cheaper. We opted to tour the Hawaiian Islands by way of our first cruise. Unfortunately, our experience didn't go as well as we had imagined, as we were visiting the islands during monsoon season and found ourselves feeling seasick at least half the time.

After our honeymoon, God continued to move and influence us. Rose was an active member at her church, and I attended services and participated in events whenever I was in town. Rose was extremely giddy when she learned about an opportunity to love and serve the less fortunate, and so we agreed to go on a mission trip to Ghana in celebration of our first wedding anniversary. It turned out to be life-changing.

I joined this mission because I had always dreamed of going to Africa, and I felt moved to use my skills to help others as God commands us to do. This trip would also allow me to see first-hand the forces of good and evil and the importance of faith and prayer. Before we left for Ghana, I gave a speech to my church congregation:

I came to accept Christ last year, and I must admit that my faith at times was not as strong as it should have been.

I recall speaking to Pastor Morgan about the cost of the trip for me and Rose. To be frank, I was concerned that we wouldn't be able to afford going because we had less than two months to raise the funds we needed. Pastor Morgan looked me straight in the eyes and said, "Wilson, you must have faith," and left it at that.

Faith, hmm, how does one have faith? Then I recalled one of Pastor Chris's sermons about having faith by praying to God. So I started praying every day, and now I would like to take this opportunity to share with you my prayer.

Lord, I put my faith in You and You alone. If you feel that this is our time to serve you, then you will provide for us. I know that at times when things aren't going our way, we lose our focus on you because we are so caught up in ourselves.

Lord, please watch over us and ensure that we are in good health so we are able to serve your purpose.

Amen.

God's hold on us was also felt by Rose. Also speaking to our church congregation, she shared the following words:

I used to think that our mission would start when we set foot on Ghanian soil, but how wrong I was.

This last month has shown me how weak I am, but more importantly, how thankful I am—thankful for a family that cares—not superficially, but with sincerity. We've had quite a few hurdles to jump over, and without your prayers, there'd be no way we'd be going to Africa…no way.

About four weeks ago, despite us having funds, we couldn't even get tickets to Ghana, let alone help the people there. My first through was, "What do you mean we can't get to Ghana? How come we can't get tickets? Were that many people dying to travel to Ghana?"

We soon realized that it wasn't to Ghana that everyone wanted to go, but to London, our connecting city. I was told that if we didn't get tickets within the week, we'd have to cancel our trip. So it was with your prayers that we found tickets for all nine of us in the next few days. Praise God for that!

The next thing that happened was a health issue—Wilson's health. Lord knows what I'd do if anything happened to him. We had a bit of a scare with his recurring neck pain. It was about this time that I felt I was falling apart. I was overwhelmed with work and with Wilson's long stays away from home. I guess I was on the verge of giving up. I was beginning to doubt God's mission for us. That was when Pastor Morgan sent me an email. He said,

"We must pray, pray and pray. We can see the spiritual warfare now. As God's children desire to serve our King, the opposition will not let us do His will that easily. Hang in there and trust the Lord!"

Once again, it was with your prayers that Wilson is as healthy as an ox, an ox with a degenerative spine, that is! Although Wilson is mostly healthy, his parents posed a bit of opposition. Needless to say, they love Wilson very much. The thought of him being in a rural village, in a developing country that is rampant with AIDS, scares them. It scares me too. So they pulled the guilt trip on me: Are these people you don't even know worth Wilson's life?

What a question. All I know is that I'm grateful for a husband who is just as passionate about serving God as I am. Wilson's parents weren't overly happy with our decision to continue to go to Ghana. It is unfortunate that we are going without their sincere blessing.

However, what amazes me most is knowing how much has happened before our departure and feeling the spirit of God moving among us. Can you imagine what it will be like when we are in Africa?

This trip would ground me and remind me to appreciate the freedom and little things I took for granted.

In an effort to reduce the cost of our trip, our one-way passage to Ghana had five layovers and took nearly twenty-seven hours. Our most memorable stop was in Addis Ababa, Ethiopia. For the first time, I had a taste of the anxiety that my parents must have felt during their exodus out of Cambodia and Vietnam. As we were waiting to board the red-eye flight to Accra, Ghana, we suddenly found ourselves in chaos. Most passengers seemed to be in a state of unrest. No one was listening to the flight attendant or following her boarding orders. People were literally pushing and shoving and making a mad dash down the runway toward the plane. We were caught in the stampede and had to run with the crowd to ensure we didn't get trampled over!

Although there is clearly no fair comparison between my parents' trek to freedom, which spanned over several years, and my meagre discomfort to just board a plane that lasted only minutes, I could not help but imagine my parents potentially caught in a similar chaotic scene, madly trying to ensure that all my siblings and I were accounted for as hordes of people left Phnom Penh because of the Khmer Rouge, or as we left Vietnam in the aftermath of the civil war. At least in my current case, the pandemonium ended once security was called and a gate was slammed shut to prevent anyone from pre-boarding the plane. Luckily, no one in our group was injured, but it was apparent that courtesy rules were not followed or honoured here.

Upon our arrival in Ghana, we were warned to keep all our luggage securely attached to us and to not accept offers from anyone to carry our baggage. Theft was fairly rampant. Sure enough, as soon as we exited the airport doors, we were hit with hot dusty air and swarms of young men who were hectoring us and trying to take our baggage from us. They left us alone as soon as they saw we had a ride with some locals.

On this trip, we were to help Reverend Joshua Siu, a pastor who had moved from Hong Kong to Ghana nearly seventeen years prior. Reverend Siu had plans to start up both a preschool and a new vocational school, specializing in computers, in Tamale. He had successfully built a school in Accra ten years earlier. But now he felt God telling him to move north.

Rose and I were definite assets to his mission. I had quite a bit of knowledge on how to fix and troubleshoot computers and networking issues, and Rose had recently graduated with her teaching certificate. Together we created a one-week course that not only focussed on tips and strategies on how to be a better teacher, but also included a hands-on component on how to address common computer issues.

Because Rose and I were the youngest couple in our group, we were invited to stay a few nights at Reverend Siu's home in the city and accompanied him on the thirteen-hour road trip to our mission site. A summer intern student from Switzerland volunteered to drive part of the way to Tamale. Unfortunately, shortly thereafter, we were stopped by the police and fined one million cedis (Ghanian currency) for excessive speeding. To be

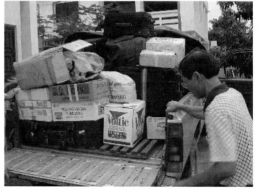

Rev. Siu loading the computer school supplies and our luggage

68

honest, I don't recall us speeding. How fast could we really have been going in a pickup truck loaded with supplies?

We had the option of paying the fine right there or travelling another seven hours from Tamale to the nearest traffic courthouse to dispute the ticket the following week. Upon hearing this, Reverend Siu immediately jumped out of the truck and began to plead with the police officer to revoke the ticket. He went on to tell him that we were on our way to build a computer school for the locals and that he had no money to pay the fine. Reverend Siu explained that he, himself, was a missionary, operating with volunteers who were only in town for a few weeks. It was then that we saw police corruption first-hand, as the officer told our pastor that he could pay a reduced fine, on the spot, for this to "all go away."

The Swiss intern, Rose and I sat dumfounded, waiting in the truck as we watched our pastor follow and plead with the officer. We decided that we would pray while we waited, as only an act of God could really change the predicament we were in. After nearly an hour, the officer let us continue on our journey, pardoning our speeding ticket. Hallelujah!

Out of our team of ten, I felt God most often put my skills to the test. I was elated and honoured, as I was here to do God's work—to be His face, hands and feet. While most of the team had opportunities to visit primary schools, enjoy street food and shop at outdoor markets in the city during our downtime, I was often asked to stay back to help set up the new lab or troubleshoot issues with the existing computer labs in Accra.

As I observed my surroundings, I felt blessed to see how happy people were with very little. It was a reminder to not get caught up with material things. I learned that one of the three female students studying with us would walk ninety minutes each way just to learn in this one-room schoolhouse, which only had the few office supplies that we had brought with us from Canada, like felt markers, tape and a stapler. We also learned that her parents had disowned her for choosing to follow Christ and not the ways of Islam. She was temporarily living with a friend, and her recent engagement had been called off.

In truth, our school was a safe place for young female students. It represented hope for them, the possibility of changing the trajectory of their lives, where they could earn a living and not just be expected to cook for their husbands and bear children. In an effort to help ease some of the stress in this particular student's life, Rose and I offered to cover her tuition for the semester, which worked out to be about US$39.

During this trip, I recognized that I had to invest in matters that came from my heart. As foreign volunteers, we were fortunate enough to stay in a multiroom home with running water and a kitchen. Our group had even brought dried and canned foods from Canada so that we could make our own meals. We had access to filtered water and made a point to regularly remind each other to take our anti-malaria medication.

To the small group of young future teachers in front of me, I was known as "Professor Wilson." It was a true honour just to be there and to be able to give them a hand up and not a handout. I was humbled and touched by the stories of each student and by the friendships I established with each of them.

But I was most in awe to witness what a true, faithful man of God looked like. Reverend Siu was truly inspiring. I couldn't imagine moving my young family and giving up everything I knew—my language, my job, the comforts of living in a developed country, which included proper health care—all because God called on me to help others. By my standards, his was a true sacrifice.

I came home to Vancouver a changed man. I began to wonder, "God, what do you want me to do? And will I be able to follow through?"

Upon our return, Rose and I participated in a church camp where we shared the details of our mission trip and recounted how God had intervened to ensure we prevailed. Upon this retelling, I began to doubt myself. How could I live up to being a 'worthy' follower of Christ? Was I doing enough?

I often felt the presence of Jesus prompting me to help and stand up for others. I always gave people the benefit of the doubt and was mindful to be a good listener. And even as I moved up the corporate/administrative ranks at work, I did my best to look out for my co-workers and to bring them up alongside me. I had such a strong desire to be God's hands and feet, and I hoped that others could see and experience God's love through me.

It was later revealed in a letter from a co-worker that others did see glimpses of God's love through my actions:

Wilson is a very supportive person. I remember attending a conference call with the office manager and the physician, both of whom were furious with us. I was upset after the conference call and felt I was not ready for this job. Wilson convinced me to give it time and gave me pointers to help me be successful. There

handle it' person. Two years into our marriage, she not only had three paying jobs—as a reading program instructor, a private tutor and a full-time schoolteacher—but she also served on the board of managers at our church and as a vocalist on the music worship team.

My frequent and extended absences for work had also distanced me from our church family. Rose told me that the only way to get us back on track was to have God be at the centre of our marriage once again. Thus, we both recommitted ourselves to prioritizing each other and our future Christ-centred family. With these measures in place, Rose terminated her private tutoring contract and began the process of leaving a ten-year, part-time job running a reading program for a private company. Little did I know that I would soon also uproot her from her beloved church family.

9

Infertility—The Dreaded 'I' Word

The original plan was to have children two years after our wedding, but my constant work trips had made it difficult for us to conceive. Rose made it very clear that she had no intentions of having a child if I continued to travel as much as I did. So within two years, I made changes to my workload and eventually fell into a position that required less out-of-town travel.

Rose was wired to do things based on a timeline. In seeing her close friends starting families of their own, she was on a mission to start ours too. Rose began to better equip herself with knowledge about ways to maximize conception. She was stocking up on ovulation sticks, tracking her menstruation cycle, improving our diet and exercising more often. This was not a new phenomenon for Rose as she was always keen to try new things, which on occasion did get quite annoying.

Shortly after we were married, I became an uncle. Holding a baby in my arms made me re-evaluate my desire and yearn more deeply to become a father. I began to think about the 'Daddy' I intended to be for my own kids.

Growing up, I often dreamed of having a more supportive father, at least someone with whom I could openly share my ideas. I didn't have a good connection with my own—we were not close. He was often at work or out enjoying himself, and when he was home, we only saw him at mealtimes. Afterwards, he would retreat into his room.

My father was traditional in every sense. He felt he was always right and knew better simply because he was older; he was not open to listening to our points of view. I saw how hard my mother worked. She held a full-time job as a seamstress and came home to cook and clean. I didn't really see my parents show love and affection for each other in the form of hugs or kisses, or even in their exchange of words. I knew that what they had wasn't true love.

In truth, my father helped me see what I didn't want to be. I wanted to be the dad that was not only the breadwinner, but also fully involved in raising his children. Furthermore, I wanted to be the loving husband who led the perfect life as portrayed in Hollywood movies. I was fortunate to have most of the pieces, now they just had to be connected.

After a year of not getting pregnant, Rose insisted that we both get full physical exams. At first, I resisted. I kept telling her I was as "healthy as an ox" and that there was nothing remotely wrong with me. However, I dreaded Rose's incessant nagging even more, and so I saw my family doctor. To my dismay, I not only suffered from low sperm count, but also learned that most of the sperm I did have were immobile due to poor morphology. I left the doctor's office in shock, my manhood completely struck. 'I' words infiltrated my mind: infertile, incompetent, impotent, immotile, insecure, incomplete. I felt so emasculated and defeated.

Why was God doing this to me?

As noted earlier, in our relationship, Rose was more of the optimist. She believed that our infertility could be overcome. So true to her character, she went on the hunt, looking to solve our predicament—low, immobile sperm. She told me that we had to investigate fertility treatments.

We spent the next three months waiting to see specialists. At the time, Rose was thirty-two. She enjoyed planning out every moment of her life, and according to her life plan, she was off-track. (She doesn't like to admit it, but she is a perfectionist and a people pleaser.)

We finally met with a urologist to see if anything could be done to improve my sperm count. After careful inspection, he told me that I had extra blood vessels, variocele, in my groin that were creating excess heat. Sperm thrive better in a cooler environment; the reason why testicles hang low on a man's body. He suggested the solution was to block these unnecessary blood vessels through a surgical procedure. Since it takes roughly three months for sperm to be produced, we would likely not see a significant change right away. Furthermore, there would be no guarantee that this surgery would solve our problem with sperm count or morphology.

At the time, we also met with another specialist, a doctor who performed in vitro fertilization (IVF) procedures. She gave us our options:

- do nothing,
- proceed with intrauterine insemination (IUI),
- fix the varicocele (excess blood vessels) and/or
- in vitro fertilization (IVF)

We wanted children, so doing nothing was not an option. Affordability was an issue for us, so we went for one round of IUI, and I was put on a wait-list for the surgery to fix my varicocele. My surgery was scheduled for six months later. Five months post-surgery, we learned that the surgery had failed—there was no change in my sperm count or morphology. We were disappointed.

In our follow-up appointment, the urologist suggested another, more invasive varicocele surgery. There would be a minor chance that my testicles would shrivel up like raisins or swell up like grapefruits. Just that notion alone scared me. But for a chance to father my own children, I was willing to take the risk. We would have to wait another six months for this next surgery.

My job still required me to be out of town, so Rose had the responsibility of following up with the surgery date. Two weeks before the operation, the urologist's office called to explain that my surgery had to be postponed due to renovations in the hospital. Rose was clearly annoyed and demanded to know when the surgery would be rescheduled. The receptionist explained that she had no idea because ours was not a life-threatening case.

Rose was tired of waiting and no longer wanted to 'put her life on hold'. In her anger, she told me to see my family doctor and demand to be referred to another urologist. Rose's exact words were, "He's not the only urologist in town. Why are we waiting for him?"

People who really know me understand that I hate redoing things or even asking for help in the first place. I really didn't want to see another medical professional, but I followed through. Looking back, this was yet another task scripted in God's plan. For when I met my new urologist, he was flabbergasted when I shared the details of my situation, saying:

> Why would they be doing your varicocele procedure at that hospital? They rarely perform that operation there. They are not as familiar as we are, since we perform these procedures here several times a month. Your surgery failed because there is still too much blood circulating to your testicles. The pieces they used to block off your vessels didn't do the job. Your sperm count is the same because the problem wasn't solved. And this new surgery? That is preposterous! Why would anyone recommend that?

With that, I had my varicocele operation redone at UBC about six months later. Although the procedure was successful in blocking the blood vessels, it didn't effectively change my sperm count or improve their morphology. Rose and I tried another unsuccessful round of IUI before deciding to put our dreams of having a baby on hold for a little while longer. In this time of waiting, Rose and I couldn't help but wonder if we were going against God's will by inviting science into the picture.

Although Rose was quite open to talking to others about our struggle to have children, we couldn't bear being around friends with young kids. It brought feelings of pain and envy. Therefore, aside from important family gatherings, we slowly phased ourselves out of spending time with anyone who had young children. This was debilitating for Rose, as she closed off relationships with her high school girlfriends. Our friend groups morphed to include single people or couples with no children.

About a year later, Rose came home from work and said she wanted to investigate IVF. She had spoken to a couple at work who had two children via IVF. They not only had no hesitations in recommending it to anyone, but they were also Roman Catholic. When Rose had mentioned her concern about going against God's will, their response was, "If God doesn't want you to have children, it won't matter what you do, you won't have any."

Who could argue with that? So off Rose went, researching and reading reviews of local IVF clinics. We ended up visiting two reputable clinics and, in doing so, were amazed to witness how many couples were also struggling with the same issues we were.

We had an instant connection with one physician. He was caring and genuinely wanted to help us. Unfortunately, the procedure would cost us about $10,000. Although we both worked full time, that was a hefty figure. In coming to this crossroad, we recognized that we needed to tell our families about our infertility and our desire to try IVF. Rose's parents instantly recognized the importance this opportunity would have for our future, so they cashed out Rose's life insurance plan, which amounted to a little over $7,000. Rose then used her extended medical coverage to cover the balance. This was a true blessing and an answer to prayer.

The IVF procedure was daunting for Rose. If all went well, we could be pregnant in about three months. She had to go through numerous tests and even a minor surgery to remove uterine fibroids to improve her chances of getting pregnant. Then, to force her body to 'super ovulate', she had to have daily injections of hormones over the course of ten days. Rose hated needles. There was no way she was going to be able to inject herself, so I was to be the one who administered these shots for her. To be honest, I secretly enjoyed those moments, watching her scream in horror from her daily hormone shot. We even filmed one injection session so I could show my future child what Mommy had to go through to have a baby.

Based on Rose's age, we expected her body to produce ten to fifteen eggs for IVF. By puberty, girls generally have about 400,000 follicles, which are fluid filled sacs that contain immature egg cells. These follicles make up the ovarian reserve. Although several follicles develop every menstrual cycle, only one mature egg is typically released into the fallopian tube each month.

To our disappointment, even with the hormone injections, Rose only had four ovarian follicles. This meant we could have at most four potential eggs to fertilize for this cycle. I say potential because not every follicle yields a viable egg. Our doctor tried to keep our spirits high by reminding us that all we needed was just one good fertilized egg.

On the day of the egg harvest, the embryologist reported that we had three "B" quality embryos. Embryos are graded on a quality scale based on their rate of development, from A to D. "A"-quality embryos are the best, with no fragmentation and even cell division. Typically, the embryos are allowed to develop in vitro, outside the womb, for up to five days, allowing the embryo to reach its blastocyst stage. At this point, our fertility clinic would update us daily about the progression of our eggs.

The next twenty-four hours were excruciatingly draining. We prayed and hoped to see signs of cell division in all the eggs. However, when we were called the next day, we were asked to return to the clinic. Only one of the eggs showed signs of cell division. And because there was only one, it was best that the embryo be put back in Rose's uterus to continue growing. This would give the embryo the best chance to survive as it would be placed in its natural environment.

Now it was the dreaded two-week waiting period. I recall it being one of the most suspenseful two weeks of our lives. We were hopeful for a child, but we were also scared of being disappointed. At the end of the two weeks, Rose went in for her blood work. We were pregnant! Hallelujah! We were over the moon! We immediately started planning for the baby.

I wanted a baby girl. I even began envisioning dancing with my daughter at her wedding to the song "Dance with My Father," by Luther Vandross. Oh, how the lyrics of this song touched me as they documented the feelings of a little girl dancing in her daddy's arms, longing for another dance when she was older after her father passes away. Little did I know that this would foreshadow my own life.

About a month later, when I was working out of town, Rose called me, crying. She was having a miscarriage. My heart sank. Although I knew my dreams of having this baby were shattering before my eyes, I couldn't imagine how much more Rose was feeling. I desperately wanted to be at her side, not just to hold her as she endured the physical loss of our child through cramping, spotting and bleeding, but moreover, I wanted to be there for her emotionally. I was immediately on the phone with a travel agent, trying to get a flight back home from the United States. Unfortunately, there were no available seats for at least two more days.

When I finally made it back home, there was an air of sadness that we couldn't shake—crushed dreams of a home without the sound and presence of children. I sat with, hugged, held and cried with Rose. For the first time in a long time, I hated my job for physically separating me from my wife in her time of need. We were in the throngs of grief.

Shortly thereafter, we had a meeting with our reproductive endocrinologist. He explained that Rose was experiencing premature ovarian aging (POA), which meant that her ovaries were aging faster than her actual age. She had a smaller ovarian reserve, meaning not only a lower quantity of eggs, but also likely eggs of poor quality. With a decline in ovarian function, it would be probable to expect a poor response to ovarian stimulation in IVF cycles. Although Rose was only thirty-four, her ovaries were acting like they were forty-five.

This diagnosis lined up with why she had had fewer eggs, despite the induced super-ovulation, and why the embryos didn't survive. The quality of her eggs were compromised. Rose had an enormous feeling of guilt—a heavy burden had been placed upon her. She liked children, but she also knew I was the one who really wanted them. Rose felt like she had let me down.

Because Rose is a fighter and a problem solver, she instinctually said, "Let's try this again!" Our doctor agreed and changed Rose's medication. He wanted to try a different superovulation cocktail—something potentially stronger. We had to wait at least three months for Rose's body to recover from the last IVF procedure before we could try again.

In this time of waiting, Rose began actively blogging about her infertility experience. She wanted prayer, and blogging would be her outlet. She also wanted to share with others her fears and desires without having to repeatedly express her pain to each person she met. This time, when we told our families about our situation, my own parents gave us $5,000 towards our next IVF procedure. We once again felt humbled and blessed to have our family stand up for us in this way.

This time, I deliberately planned my travel schedule to ensure I was home for the entire process. When it came time to harvest the eggs, Rose had four follicles and the same number of viable eggs as last time—three. After fertilization, once again there was only one viable, fertilized egg. We hoped for another blessing—a baby in nine months. Unfortunately, Rose miscarried at the end of the two-week waiting period. We were both devastated.

During our follow-up appointment, it was clear that we would not be able to conceive on our own. Rose doesn't cry often, but the reality of our situation caused her eyes to well up incessantly. I pleaded with the doctor to let us to try IVF one more time. He said,

> If I just wanted your money, I would say, "Yes." But the outcome will be the same. You need an egg donor. In Canada, someone must voluntarily be your egg donor. But if you don't have a donor, I can help set you up to find and pay for one in Seattle. You would be looking at an additional $10,000 for an egg donor. The whole procedure would also have to be done at a clinic in Seattle. You would be looking at spending about $30,000.

Rose was quiet. It was a lot to take in. What was God telling us? Yes or no? Rose looked at me and then at the doctor. She shook her head and said, "No. No egg donor."

I remember our fertility doctor looking intently at Rose as tears were streaming down her face. "Rose, don't close the door on this. I have a feeling I will see you in the future."

It was eerily quiet in our house for the next few days. I spent a lot of time in front of the TV, and Rose was often at her computer. It was summer, so she wasn't working. She told me later that she spent her days reading other people's blogs and looking up alternative solutions. She was also praying a lot, although to me it looked like she was just talking and crying a lot to God.

It was clear to me that, in her pain, Rose leaned more on God. But that wasn't how I felt. I harboured innate anger. As I grew angrier at God, she drew closer to Him. To a certain extent, I resented her. How could she continue onward? Why was she not consumed by disappointment and resentment like I was?

Rose continued to pray. A few days later, she approached me to say,

Honey, I know you really want your 'own' kids. Although it breaks my heart to think that we can't have children that are genetically both of ours, my genetics coursing through our children is really not that important to me. I've always envisioned us adopting. If not that, what about using donor eggs like our doctor suggested? I know I was initially dead set against it, but I've been asking God a lot of things recently. I'm thinking about asking my younger sister to help us. In Canada, we have to provide our own egg donor. If my sister agrees, our child will still have some of my genetics and all of yours. It seems like the best solution at this point in time.

With careful thought, I was totally on board with this idea. Rose called her sister, who said without hesitation, "Of course I will help you!" Although we were ecstatic, we both knew that this would complicate the story we would have to tell our child as he or she grew up. Who was their biological mother? Yes, Rose would carry the baby to term, and we would raise him or her, but from a genetics standpoint, wouldn't my sister-in-law be the biological mother? How and when do we explain that to our child? Rose was very anxious about telling my family. How would we ensure other family members did not jump the gun and tell our child before we did?

Also, Rose's sister was in a relationship. Would her partner be okay with this? Then we had Rose's mom, who was adamant about keeping this all a secret. Her viewpoint: "Why are you making things so complicated? It's not necessary for your child to know that they came from their aunt's egg. Rose is his/her mother. End of story." There were so many questions, and Rose was clearly stressed by the whole ordeal. We disagreed with her mom's point of view. We didn't want our child to grow up without knowing their true roots. No life should be based on the foundation of a lie, no matter how small. We sought professional help to field all these questions.

We entered our next fertility cycle with mixed feelings of anxiety and excitement. Rose and her sister were taking medications to synchronize their menstrual cycles. As the egg harvesting day approached, regular transvaginal ultrasounds were taken to monitor the development of the eggs. Unfortunately, Rose and her sister had the same genetic predisposition. Based on the ultrasounds, both sisters suffered from premature ovarian aging. Despite her sister being nearly seven years younger, she, like Rose, only had a few good-sized antral follicles.

In an effort to harvest the follicles at their optimal size, which would be our best chance at obtaining mature eggs, our doctor suggested we wait one more day. Unfortunately, when we returned the next day, the follicles were now too large. Due to the intricacies and complexity of egg cells, eggs that are retrieved from follicles that are too large have a reduced ability to implant in the uterus, thus rendering the eggs potentially useless. Our cycle had to be cancelled.

We took this as God's message, advising us that this was not His will. We were not going to have children using my sister-in-law's eggs. I'd be lying if I told you I wasn't disappointed.

In fact, this is when my life took an abrupt turn. The emotional walls that I had carefully built to protect myself all came crashing down like a ton of bricks. I began to unravel and self-destruct. I couldn't sleep, so for the first time in my adult life, I took a short-term leave of absence from work. I didn't want to eat, and I couldn't focus. This would be the first of many lessons God put in front of me, teaching me to drop my pride and sense of entitlement.

In the beginning, I had taken time off to be at home with Rose—to be her comforter. But as it turned out, God needed me to face my own reality. I spun my anger into a massive demon. I noticed that my uncontrollable temper had come back. I was not nice to be around. I felt like it was my fault for having faulty sperm. I began analyzing my life. Was this a side effect of my fall in Thailand? Was this the trade-off? My life for a future with no kids? This wasn't fair to Rose. I blamed myself. I knew she would be a great mother, and I felt responsible for not giving her that opportunity. I also wanted Rose's parents to be grandparents. I was disappointing them too.

I found myself turning away from both God and Rose. I blamed Him for my predicament. If He is the Great I Am, why couldn't He just perform a miracle for us? I thought, "Why? Why me, God? Why do I have to struggle for everything? How is this fair? Do you not love me? What have I done wrong to deserve this? This is not the future I promised Rose."

As I cried out in agony, I just got more upset. My rants to God continued: "Why am I cursed to suffer? Why am I so unlucky? Have I not already suffered enough? Why are undeserving people—adults who are not good role models—becoming parents and not me? Why are people aborting babies while I struggle through the pain of multiple miscarriages? How is Joe Schmoe, who doesn't even want a child, blessed with one or more? How are they more deserving than me? God, are you even there? Do you even exist? If so, why are my non-Christian friends, who are clearly not making sound moral choices, enjoying all the things of this world?"

In my lashing out, I decided to abandon God: "I don't need you!"

I didn't need Him. It seemed that everything I had was accomplished by my own accord, my own perseverance and my own blood, sweat and tears.

I hurled into a clinical depression. Preliminary signs of my deteriorating mental health started showing shortly after Rose's first miscarriage. I was broken then, but by now, with God showing me that no baby would be in my future, I was beyond devastated. This baby had symbolized my hope, my future, my legacy. I desperately wanted to be the father I never had. I had so much love to offer. Why was God denying me this opportunity?

It soon became even more difficult for Rose and me to be around anyone welcoming their little ones. As happy as we were for them, it just reminded us of what we couldn't have. It was too painful and too hard to disguise our agony with smiles and words of joy—so we distanced ourselves from them.

My family doctor soon prescribed me a mild anti-depressant and sleeping pills to deal with my mood and restlessness. Rose more or less left me alone these few months. She tried her best to feed me and talk with me. Because I spent a lot of time binge-watching various Chinese and American TV series, she would regularly join me on the couch to watch a few episodes of whatever I was watching. But in truth, I didn't want to be around her either. I had to shut her out because I felt that I had failed her and that my life was meaningless.

I soon found that watching hours on end of TV was no longer soothing enough. I started going to movie theatres on my own in an effort to block my mind from feeling sad. But soon that too wasn't enough, so I began gambling. It started off small, just a group of friends playing poker for fun. Soon, some of my single friends decided it would be more 'exciting' to play sexually provocative videos in the background. This then escalated to hiring 'sexy' female card dealers. They continued to up the ante. These poker nights moved from being casual games at a friend's house to nights out in Whistler with hired escorts.

In all honesty, I went to these outings to play poker. I figured that since I wasn't physically cheating on Rose, it was okay to be there. After all, I reasoned to myself, it would look bad to my friends if I stopped showing up to these parties because my wife didn't like it. At the time, I didn't take into consideration that even my attendance was contributing to a system that was degrading to women. In retrospect, I was getting a taste of Sodom and Gomorrah.

I ignored my friends' 'words of wisdom', telling me to keep my mouth shut about our poker nights. I called Rose when I finally found out just how far the boys were going to take things to keep our poker games entertaining. Needless to say, Rose was pissed. I can count on my fingers how many heated arguments we have had in our many years together. This was one of them. My very presence there had crossed the line. In her anger, frustration and disappointment, she slammed the phone down on me. I left the game, as the boys shook their heads and called me 'stupid', and drove straight home to Rose.

Yes, I was coming home to a very upset wife. But we always worked things out, even if it meant a few days of the cold shoulder or silent treatment. As much as I told Rose how much I loved her, she didn't understand how deeply I had attached myself to her. I couldn't bear the thought of hurting or losing her. I had vowed to always be open and honest with her, even if it meant her being angry with me. If I gave her my word, I stuck to it.

Rose asked me if it had been worth it, and in the back of my mind, I secretly feared she would leave me. I knew what kind of a man she deserved. I promised to stop attending these 'unclean' poker games.

But I still had a void in my life—a hole that desperately needed to be filled. So I started going to local casinos a few times a month. Soon the frequency increased to a few times a week and then, at my peak, almost daily. I would gamble into the wee hours of the night. Eventually, Rose stepped in and limited my time at the casino, but I just picked up online gambling instead. We began to have heated arguments over my addiction. Of course, I didn't see it as an addiction. I always told Rose I was in control.

I did eventually put limits on my credit card, just to give Rose a sense of security that I wouldn't drive us into debt. I managed to pull myself together enough to go back to work, but Rose soon became concerned with my health. I wasn't sleeping well, and I didn't want to rely on medications. I continued gambling and I wanted nothing to do with God. I just wanted to blow money.

As I was dealing with my demons, I would later learn that Rose had been spending her time trying to find a path forward for our childless family—adoption. Once she was hung up on an idea, she would push her agenda until I could give her a valid reason as to why it wouldn't work. Her exact words: "Let's adopt. I don't need to be pregnant. There are perfectly good kids who need homes with great parents. We can look internationally. This way, we don't run the risk of birth parents wanting to be a part of our child's life. I was thinking about a Southeast Asian country like Thailand. Yes, I know HIV is rampant there. We will just need to ensure the child we adopt is healthy."

That's one of the things about Rose. She doesn't outright 'ask', she just tells you what she wants. I had no interest in adopting, so I simply replied, "No. I would rather not have any kids, Rose."

"What's so special about your sperm?" she said. "What's so special about your genetic material that you feel you have to pass that on? You realize you would pass on this infertility problem to a son, right? Why wouldn't you love your adopted child as much as your own biological one? Do you not love our dog? Just think about how much we love Tiger. I didn't give birth to him. And it goes both ways. Tiger clearly loves us, and we didn't give birth to him!"

I knew what she said made some sense, but my heart couldn't let it go. I kept telling her it wasn't the same. I couldn't get past my own demons. I wanted to see my genetic traits and my bloodline coursing through my child. I wanted to be a part of the birthing experience. I wanted to see my child growing in Rose's belly, and I wanted to be in the delivery room when my child took their first breath.

At first, I thought my aversion to adoption was due to my sense of pride and manhood. But later I realized, I felt entitled to be a biological parent. It was my right, wasn't it? I worked hard. I was honest. I was nice. I even showed generosity and treated homeless people to lunch once in a while. Why was life so unfair? How was God just?

As I saw my anger intensify, I saw the complete opposite in Rose. She grew stronger in her faith. She told me that she was strengthened by God's presence. In fact, she later disclosed to me that God had assured her that she would be a parent. She said, "God tells me that we will have three children in our lives. He tells me not to worry. I will be a parent."

I didn't really understand her relationship with God. "What do you mean, God 'told' you? How do you know?"

She was quiet and shrugged her shoulders. "I just feel it."

To be honest, this made me resent her even more. Why was God talking to her and answering her prayers? Why not me?

Rose convinced me that I had to see a psychologist. In actuality, it was more like an ultimatum. I remember telling her, "What good is it to tell someone else my problems? What can they do about it? It's such a waste of my time, and I have to pay for it!"

Rose's response: "I will pay for it, and I will go with you."

She knew that I would procrastinate, and also that we needed a referral from my family doctor. Rose's take-care-of-business attitude kicked in, and she went with me to see my GP to ensure we walked out of the doctor's office with the name of a psychologist. I was not a willing participant—in fact, I wanted no part of this. I was doing this just to appease her. This was yet another reason to resent her.

I vividly recall that first meeting with the psychologist. I might have said three sentences in that one-hour session. Rose did almost all the talking. In retrospect, that first session helped me a lot, as I had an opportunity to listen to Rose share her side of the story. Up until that point, I really only knew bits and pieces of what she had experienced and a small fraction of the depth of her own pain. I had often wondered how she remained so calm. That's when I heard her tell the therapist that God was her source of strength.

I attended two more sessions on my own. Rose was not allowed to be a part of those sessions, to ensure that I could be open and honest, allowing for moments where I could learn more about myself. In keeping an open mind, I realized why I was so hung up on having my own 'bloodline' of descendants. I wanted to be everything my father wasn't. I wanted to tell my children that I loved them. I wanted to be supportive, present—a mentor. I wanted to have a close relationship with my children, like what I saw in the movies.

I wanted to reciprocate a love that I felt was missing in my childhood. I wanted to be there for every moment of their lives, to experience their firsts—first steps, first words, first day of school, first boyfriend/girlfriend, etc. I wanted to be there in their darkest times to not only express my love to them, but also to show them how to persevere and face their problems. I wanted to provide opportunities for them. I wanted them to be proud of their daddy! How ironic that all sounds now.

In essence, I wanted to love a part of me in the way that I had always wanted to be loved. I also wanted to receive for myself this unconditional love that I felt for my father. Although I knew I was loved unconditionally by God, I couldn't feel it. I couldn't see past my anger and wasn't open to feeling and seeing His love working through others in my life.

Although these sessions with the psychologist helped me see the root of my pain, I wasn't able to see past it enough to feel the grace and value of this life God had blessed me with. I still couldn't see past my sense of entitlement. I felt God was unfair. I grew bitter, and I began to lash out.

Despite my position on adoption, Rose had secretly been working on getting the paperwork together for the adoption agency. She said, "I know you are not keen on adopting, but I'd really like to adopt a child overseas. There is an agency in Kelowna that is working on baby adoptions from Taiwan. They could match us up with a teen mom. This agency is only in the preliminary stages of starting this program. I have already filled out the application form for us. I will submit the paperwork when you feel you are ready for this next step."

I was annoyed. Why was she doing this? She knew that I didn't want to adopt. I responded, "Whatever. You can wait forever then."

I continued on my downward trend of self-loathing and self-pity. It was me against the world. I threw myself back into gambling at casinos, both on- and offline. I also began spending, buying things I didn't need with money we really didn't have. I self-indulged and splurged, and I didn't consult Rose about any of it. In just a short period of time, I bought a new car, an expensive watch, a new TV—essentially any new electronics on the market. (Among the slew of things I did that were bad for my relationships, for my body and for my mind, I also developed a few good ones, like my love of raising fish.)

Soon I began to give in to all my wants. I was trapped by the Seven Deadly Sins. The Lord tells us to treat our body like His temple, but in my anger and disappointment toward Him, where I saw my future with no children of my own, I didn't feel I had to follow His ways. I started to eat more recklessly, abusing my body in the process—gluttony. I began go on binges where I would eat two or three large beef burgers, a family pack of fried chicken, containing eight to ten pieces, or a dozen Krispy Kreme donuts, all in one sitting. I would frequently overindulge with steak and lobster dinners. In doing these things, I gained a substantial amount of weight. So much so that my GP had to prescribe me medications to control my rising sugar and cholesterol levels. I was soon also diagnosed with sleep apnea.

I found myself always wanting things that I didn't need—greed. I was constantly trying to buy more fish for my tanks or upgrade my electronics. I chased the momentary feelings of happiness that new objects could give me.

I succumbed to hours spent binge-watching Chinese or American TV series—sloth. I refused to leave the house unless it was to eat or to see certain members of my family. I had clearly lost all desire to take care of myself and to treat my life as a gift and my body as a temple for God.

10

God's Grace and Miracle

In response to my depression and my unwillingness to adopt, my mother and aunt suggested we try Chinese medicine to improve our chances to conceive naturally. We figured we had nothing to lose.

Rose and her mom spent four to six hours every week making these nasty herbal concoctions that Rose and I would each drink daily. We stuck to this regimen for at least three months before finally throwing in the towel. We also committed to eating healthy and exercising more so that we could be in better shape to try another attempt at the IUI procedure. We wanted to leave no stone unturned, no excuse to say we didn't try every possible option. My parents even went to seek counsel from a few fortune tellers to see if there was anything else we could do to improve our odds of getting pregnant.

It was clear that I had lost my way in this past year. But God knew that in my heart I was still tethered to Him, and as signs of my depression subsided, my anger toward God softened. I didn't hate Him, but I wasn't quite ready to commit to regularly going to church.

Rose remained a faithful church attendee. Once in a while, I would take her up on the offer to join her, just to surprise her. But I soon started to revert to my old ways, putting work before everything else. Rose began to question my hesitancy at attending church service, often reminding me about our spiritually rewarding time in Ghana, saying, "I go to worship God and to grow in my faith with others. You can't do that on your own. If you dislike our current church community that much, let's find a new one. I need us to be united again."

So here we were, church hopping once again. Admittedly, this time I was not as motivated as Rose. But we did finally find a faith community that resonated with us, and before committing to them, I asked Rose to promise me not to pour all of her extra time into serving this place of worship.

We compromised and began to work on rebuilding our relationship. We started travelling more. Because of my job, I had a significant number of air miles, car rental and hotel points. Rose would sometimes join me on my business trips, and we planned at least one international vacation every year. Over the course of a few short years, we visited the Caribbean Islands, Greece, Italy and parts of Asia. I savoured these vacations with Rose as I had a chance to really relax my mind and enjoy spending time with my wife.

It was after returning from one of our vacations that Rose decided she didn't want to waste any more time thinking about children. She had started to imagine a life without them and had begun to ponder all the things she had put on hold over the last seven years in our efforts to start a family.

Rose started attending a small Christian study group and eventually started hosting weekly church life meetings in our home. That's when she told me she was going to Cambodia on a medical mission trip with 'her' church—with or without me.

Rose was gone for almost three weeks. Because she was volunteering in remote villages, we could only communicate by email when she had access to Wi-Fi. In her absence, I attended a friend's wedding on my own and had a lot of time to really reflect on my values. I was forced to deal with the silence of my home and to address my relationship with God. I slowly began singing and listening to music, reading and writing poems again. I even wrote a letter/poem to God that I shared with Rose in one of our email exchanges.

I realized how much I missed her presence, and that was when I had my epiphany—she was enough. I didn't need kids. This was God's lesson to me: Be happy with the gifts I have put forth before you.

Lord, it is no surprise that I have fallen from your grace.
I feel that you've abandoned me during my greatest time of need.
Therefore, I've made a conscious choice to abandon you!
>   I know all the stories of tribulation and triumph.
>   But Lord, is this pain really necessary?
>   To give me such great hope
>   that fills my heart to its brim.
>   Then to rip it away so viciously…
>   without regard
>   without hope.

Lord, it's been over a year and yet the pain is still here.
Is time not supposed to heal all wounds?
I am still waiting for that moment when I can live again.
I still can't talk about it as my emotions overwhelm me.
I weep to myself in secret like a thief afraid to get caught.
I wish I was as strong as Rose, as I know her suffering is
>   much greater. I hate that I am so weak, and yet I can't do
>   anything about it.

Father, I have so much love in my heart that it's going to burst.
And yet I fear it like the plague.
Lord, I hear YOU calling me, and yet I choose to ignore YOU
>   because I am afraid.
I am afraid because I am damaged goods.
Therefore, I can't see how I can help.
I am afraid because I might forget that feeling I had experienced
>   when Rose was pregnant. I am afraid that I might forget her
>   altogether….

Father, as I pour out my heart to you, I hope you can take this
FEAR away.
>   Father, as I pour my soul to you, I hope that you will forgive me.
>   Father, as I pour my tears to you, I hope that you can heal me.
>   Father, as I pour my pain to you, I hope that you will take it away.
>   Father…Father, please forgive me for I know not what I
have done.
>   Father, please live in me again...

>   — *Wilson Ngo*
>   *July 29, 2011*

Rose's trip to Cambodia was orchestrated so that she, too, could reconcile with God. When she came home, we agreed that it was time for us to turn a new leaf. God performs miracles. If our story included a biological child, then one would come. It would not be by our will, but through His.

Nearly a year later, in the summer of 2012, on the last night of our first church retreat just outside of Bellingham, Washington, I told Rose I was ready to adopt a child overseas. I'll never forget the look on her face. She was beaming. "You have no idea how long I have waited to hear those words!"

Rose quickly contacted the agency she had been working with, only to find that the program had never opened. She started contacting other adoption agencies in the lower mainland of British Columbia and met up with a relative of ours who had adopted her two girls overseas. Shortly thereafter, we attended an informational session at an adoption agency and met with a social worker for a consultation.

To our dismay, the agency told us that there were fewer children up for adoption this year than in previous years. One reason for this decrease was that more families in many of these southeast Asian countries could now, with lower rates of unemployment coupled with sex education outreach and access to contraceptives, afford to raise their own children. Another reason for fewer adoptees was due to bureaucracy. There were a significant number of children still waiting for their papers to be processed. On top of this, the cost of international adoption had nearly doubled from two years prior, to upwards of $40,000 when you factored in travel costs. Aside from not having the money to adopt, from our standpoint, three to five years' wait time was unacceptably long. We left that meeting dejected.

Rose was infinitely more disappointed than I was. She came home extremely confused and kept repeating, "I thought this was the plan, God! If not this, then what?"

God had clearly slammed the door shut in our faces, so we dropped our thoughts of pursuing children. Rose instead began to dream about what we could do to change the world. I started to attend more church services and agreed to be a part of a church life group.

About six months later, at our family's New Year's dinner, my aunt told me about a relative in Vietnam who was using a surrogate from Thailand to have their child. My aunt and I had never personally spoken about my difficulty in having children. I knew this was a sign from God.

Rose and I both agreed that we didn't need a surrogate to carry our baby, but we wondered if a similar clinic might offer donor eggs and at what price. Rose made it very clear that if we were to go down this road, this would be her "last kick at the IVF can," as she had entitled her latest blog.

To our surprise, I found two reputable IVF clinics in Thailand. To ensure we weren't being scammed, we had my boss's girlfriend, who lived in Thailand, check out both locations. She told us that both clinics were legitimate businesses that dealt strictly with international clients. The cost, including donor eggs, was the same price as an IVF cycle performed locally, about $10,000. We decided that if the IVF procedure didn't work, we would at least have a vacation in Thailand.

I was extremely anxious and excited as the details of the plan played out. Rose began taking medications to synch up her cycle with that of the donor's, and we shared our IVF venture with a few of our close friends and family so we could receive prayer for this new chapter in our journey for children.

Once in Thailand, both Rose and I tried our best to keep an open mind while also guarding our hearts, knowing that we might not get pregnant despite the use of an egg donor. We did our best to enjoy the sights and beauty around us, but it was hard. In the back of our minds, we knew that this was our last chance at becoming biological parents.

Everything about our international IVF experience was amazing. We were stunned by how many couples, of various ages, faiths, ethnic backgrounds and sexual orientation, were in the clinic's waiting room with us. We were all here for one thing—the hope for a child to call our own.

Normally, egg donors do not meet recipients in order to preserve anonymity, but Rose really wanted to share her gratitude with her donor. God made all the stars align, and we did get to meet her, and although our donor did not speak much English, words weren't needed. She understood how grateful we were as she watched tears stream down Rose's face from the moment we were introduced.

Our donor blessed us with fourteen eggs, three of which were AA quality. Once the eggs were removed from the donor, my sperm was used to fertilize them. We knew most people transferred two eggs because often only one egg makes it to full term. Because Rose had no intention of getting pregnant again, we really hoped for twins. We didn't believe in gender selection, but we secretly hoped for one boy and one girl.

With our hopes in mind, I asked our doctor if all three AA eggs could be transferred to Rose's womb. The doctor immediately objected.

He said that given the quality of the eggs, we would likely have triplets, leading to a high-risk pregnancy. (There was also a small chance we could have triplets by just transferring two eggs!) It was risky to carry twins, let alone triplets, so we heeded the doctor's advice and transferred only two eggs.

The dreaded two-week waiting period was upon us yet again. We faced it with a mixture of anxiety and hope. In my paranoia, I made sure Rose only participated in outings that required minimal physical effort, strength or endurance. We took one final blood test two weeks later before heading back home to Canada. Our HCG levels were through the roof. Hallelujah! We were likely pregnant with twins!

We cautiously savoured the next few months. I say "we" because I felt like I was actively a part of the pregnancy experience. I seemed to have unexplained cravings, strangely more that Rose did! But being pregnant with twins made life physically tough on Rose. She gained over fifty pounds and was on bedrest after her second trimester. She suffered from morning sickness every day, for eight months, until our babies were born.

During her pregnancy, we also sold our home, and thus I took on the brunt of dealing with the stresses of a move. I helped Rose as best as I could by trying to keep things lighthearted. We continued to have our date nights, and I would often make fun of her swollen feet as I helped her put on her shoes. I was so excited to meet the twins.

The happiest day of my life—correction, the second happiest day of my life—was when the twins were born. I had been waiting for this moment to meet my 'mini mes' for what seemed like an eternity. Rose and I planned to share the twelve-month parental leave. We would both be off work during the first month to really enjoy being new parents, then Rose would take the following ten months to be home with them while I returned to work. I would then take another leave from work just before they turned one, to not only enjoy the twins on my own, but also to establish caregiver routines for both sets of grandparents once Rose and I were back at work full-time.

I could hardly contain myself when Rose called me from the washroom while I was watching TV in our tiny bedroom. She said, "I think my water broke."

Alarm bells went off. I had practiced this moment in my mind, but now I was lost! We had a scheduled C-section for the following week. I stared at Rose with a blank face. She looked straight at me and calmly told me to call the hospital. I could barely speak; my words were jumbled. Rose told me to pass her the phone.

We had moved in with my in-laws while we were between homes, and Rose's sister had just come home from work when we got off the phone. We filled her in, and the three of us headed to the hospital together.

Rose had decided beforehand that she wanted to give birth naturally. I told her it wasn't a good idea, but she had been reading up about it and really wanted to give it a go. I went along with her plan.

We arrived at the hospital around six o'clock. The nurses gave her oxytocin at nine o'clock, as Rose was still only one centimetre dilated. Over the next fifteen hours, Rose was in constant and extreme discomfort. Despite my messaging her neck and shoulders, the cramping would not relent. Furthermore, her cervix would not dilate past four centimetres. I remember not feeling well myself as I watched the nurses prep her epidural. I was glad that it wasn't me getting a large needle inserted into my spine.

At noon the next day, our obstetrician arrived and told Rose that it was time to go for the C-section. Rose was grateful for the opportunity to try to give birth naturally but was relieved that she wouldn't have to endure any more pain or wait any longer to see her twin babies. They wheeled her into the operating room, and I suited up before sitting down next to an exhausted but calm Rose. We were ready to meet our twins.

As the medical team put up the curtain, the anesthetist gave Rose some medication to numb her from the waist down. I could tell that Rose was now a bit on edge, as giving birth had been a great fear for her. She did not have a high tolerance for pain and couldn't fathom how she could deliver two babies. When the OB/GYN (obstetrician/gynecologist) stepped in and started drawing on her belly, Rose began to freak out. She exclaimed, "Am I supposed to be able to feel your pen strokes?"

The overall feeling in the room was no longer one of calm. Her obstetrician quickly replied, "You can feel my pen strokes?" Rose nodded her head. The panic set in as she began to imagine herself feeling every incision the OB/GYN would soon make. There was a flurry of action, and I was quickly escorted out of the delivery room and told to wait outside. Rose was to be 'put under' using a general anesthetic. I was disappointed I wouldn't be able to cut the twins' umbilical cords, but it was more important to me that everyone was safe.

I anxiously waited outside of the operating room for what seemed like an eternity. I was overcome with so many emotions. At one point, I saw a frenzy of doctors and nurses running in and out of Rose's room. My heart froze. Something was wrong.

One of the doctors noticed my panic-stricken face and told me that everything was under control. I would be able to see the twins and Rose once they were in recovery. As I continued to wait in the hallway, I overheard one of the doctors saying that the babies were not breathing. I knew a team was madly resuscitating my twins. Isabella, my eldest, a precious baby girl, woke up taking her first independent breaths after five minutes, and Isaac, my beloved baby boy, took his first independent breaths twelve minutes post-delivery. The fantastic NICU (neonatal intensive care unit) medical team had been helping my babies breathe until they woke, minimizing any brain damage.

Shortly thereafter, our OB/GYN came out and congratulated me, telling me my twins were fine and that I could now see them. I was excited and truly grateful that my twins were alive and well, especially after such an emotional delivery. But at that point, I blurted out the one thing that was running through my mind, "What about my wife?"

A nurse called me into the recovery room as Rose was waking up from the anaesthesia. She was semi-conscious and had no idea I was in the room with her. Doctors and nurses were continually coming in, massaging and feeling her uterus to help it contract post-delivery. I stepped out to use the washroom, and as I returned to the ward, I heard Rose screaming. I quickly ran to her only to be met by what I can best describe as a scene in a horror movie. I saw my wife screaming as a steady stream of blood and tissue exited her body. Rose was hemorrhaging, and a doctor was doing what he could to manually remove blood clots from her uterus. Once again, I was quickly told to leave the room. There was nothing to do but wait in the hallway.

Over the course of her C-section and subsequent hemorrhage, Rose lost almost 1.3 litres of blood, a bit more than one-fourth of the blood in her body. Thankfully, no blood transfusion was necessary, but she was kept in the ICU for the next day so she could be monitored closely.

While Rose was resting, I doted on the two new loves of my life—my twins. I couldn't contain my joy. I called my closest family members and friends to visit us at the hospital. Rose met our twins about seven hours after they were born. Since she was still weak from the surgery and the uterine hemorrhage, she didn't have the strength to carry them. But because it is so important that newborns have skin-to-skin contact with their mother, the nurse and I gently placed each twin against her chest. Rose later described the moment as unbelievably perfect.

On Sunday, March 16, 2014, Rose and the twins finally came home after spending a week in the hospital. It was a magical moment leaving the hospital with not just a wife, but also with two newborn babies in the back seat. It was surreal. I had been dreaming of this moment for years, and now I was living it. I was giddy, anxious and excited just to be driving home from the hospital! I did my best to be supportive and involved. I set my alarm to remind us of their feeding times. We would both wake up to feed them, alternating between breast milk and infant formula. I changed diapers, helped bathe them and ran errands. Throughout the day and into the evening, Rose and I would often just sit and watch the twins sleep, taking in the fact that we had finally made it. Parenthood.

Just four days after being discharged from the hospital, Rose noticed that she was passing blood clots. At first, they were small, but by Friday the clots were not only increasing in size but also in frequency. At eleven o'clock Saturday night, Rose stepped out of the washroom to let me know that the clots weren't letting up, and she thought it best if she just sat on the toilet for a while. She took the iPad with her to look up information about postpartum hemorrhaging. I heard her call out for me. She was having trouble breathing, feeling light-headed and she was in a cold sweat. She told me to call 911.

After doing so, I called Rose's sister to come downstairs and asked her to not only help direct the paramedics to us in the washroom, but to also go with Rose to the hospital. As much as I wanted to go with them, I had to stay at home to take care of the twins. By the time the ambulance arrived, Rose was shivering uncontrollably. The paramedics had trouble just getting the IV into her arm.

It was an awful night. I felt alone—abandoned, even—and felt the weight of the world was on my shoulders. I thought, "What if Rose doesn't make it home? How can I raise these two on my own?" The answer was that I couldn't.

God was at the forefront of my mind again. "Lord, you can't do this to me! Take me, Lord, not her. The twins for her? No! This was not the deal. I can't imagine my life without her. The pain would be too much. Lord, you said you wouldn't take me where you couldn't sustain me. Lord, I am telling you, I won't make it."

Between feeding the twins and getting updates from my sister-in-law about Rose's progress, I didn't get much sleep that night. In desperation, I wept as I called my mother and sisters early that morning for their help in taking care of the twins so that I could visit Rose at the hospital.

By the time I saw Rose, she had lost so much blood that she had needed a blood transfusion. The doctors informed me that she had likely contracted a bacterial infection in her uterus from attempting to deliver vaginally. Amazingly, God made sure Rose's GP was in the hospital each time she was admitted to the ER, so I knew she was in good hands.

When Rose came home after spending a few nights in the hospital, I was reminded of the precious gift of life and the presence of God. We resumed our lives, learning how to balance taking care of the twins and each other. I planned regular outings with Rose in which we enjoyed watching movies and dining out either as a family or with friends. We often brought our twins with us, though they mostly slept in their carriers next to us.

We stayed at my in-laws' for a few months as we transitioned from one home to another. And although it was great staying with my mother-in-law, and we were so appreciative of the extra help, it was also a stressful time for us as I was overseeing the building of our new home. I wanted everything to be perfect. For my own mental well-being, I arranged family road trips to Whistler and Seattle. My parents and siblings thought I was crazy to plan for such events with my infant twins, but I wanted my babies to experience my joy and happiness in a vacation setting.

It wasn't until we moved in and settled into our new home, with our now seven-month-old twins, that I felt my life was complete. For the first time in a long while, I felt whole. My life was essentially perfect.

I made every effort to be at home and be present for my twins. Rose and I were a great tag team. I loved going out with the twins. They made me feel proud and grateful to be a father. We'd either each carry a child in a cloth baby carrier or push the two of them in their double stroller. When I was home, I helped to feed them, regularly prepping baby formula and waking up with Rose for their scheduled feedings.

We all loved bath times together. I had a fantastic set-up for bathing them in their infant tub. Then as they grew bigger, I was the one sitting in the larger tub, helping them sit up, gently washing, rinsing and playing with them. Once I was done, Rose would dry and dress them.

I loved watching them sleep, and hearing them giggle melted my heart. I'd often crawl around on all fours or just lie next to them for hours. I'd swing them, toss them in the air and catch them. I'd sing sappy love songs, kiss them on their necks and blow raspberries on their little tummies.

While Rose opted to go back to work when the twins were ten months old, I spent an extra month on parental leave with my little ones. I had the added luxury of having both sets of grandparents babysit during this time, since my role was to help the twins transition from being cared for by us to being cared for by our parents.

Once I was back at work, and the twins had settled into their new routine with the grandparents, I began to realize the importance of having a work/life balance. I made sure that I spent time playing with my babies and was present to see them hit milestones in their development, like their first solid foods, their first walks and first words. I enjoyed making faces and being the 'patient', receiving a shot from a pretend needle from Doctor Bella. I routinely shared candies with Isaac and lovingly bit his cute bum.

I also loved dressing up in matching father–son outfits with Isaac. A classic example would be both of us sporting identical golf shirts and shorts. As the twins got older, we would sit and watch TV together. I made it a habit of putting the twins to sleep by singing at least one song, setting up background music and praying for them. I held their little hands until they fell asleep.

When the twins were fifteen months old, Rose decided that she wanted to undergo elective surgery to correct her diastasis recti, or the significant separation between the left and right abdominal muscles as a result of pregnancy. This meant she would be on bedrest for six to eight weeks. Although Rose arranged for her sister to stay with us for two months, this meant I would have to take the lead in caring for the twins. It was during these six weeks that I really learned how much work went into being an attentive parent. I had to not only feed, play with, change, bathe and put the twins to bed, but also help Rose get in and out of bed because of the stitches on her abdomen.

I tend to be someone who likes to be spontaneous, flying by the seat of my pants. I learned very quickly that I couldn't parent twin toddlers on my own with that kind of a mindset. Rose showed me how she scheduled her day. It included meal planning, cleaning, playing, reading, etc. I recall looking at her plan and telling her, "No way! I'm going to do it my way. When you are better, you can go back to doing it your way. I'm just making sure we are fed and that the kids stay alive."

I felt completely burned out by the end of Rose's eight-week recovery. This was also when I began to realize I wasn't feeling quite right.

11

A Death Sentence?

When Rose was pregnant, my eating habits were pretty poor. I took the liberty to binge-eat sweets and meat, jokingly telling others that I was also "eating for two." Even though we were living at Rose's parents' place, I didn't feel the need to eat what my mother-in-law cooked, especially since she predominately cooked vegetables. As rude as it looked, if I didn't find what was on the table appetizing, I ordered takeout.

After the twins were born, I now had new excuses to cover up my weight gain. I told others that I was busy caring for the twins and that I was quite stressed at work. Over the previous years, work had been creeping back into my personal life, and my current workplace was no longer a joyful one. The relationships I had at work seemed rather superficial. I was not happy, and it showed.

When Rose recovered from her post-pregnancy surgery to bridge the gap between her abdominal muscles, I began to notice a change in my bowel activity. I had always prided myself on 'going' twice a day, usually after each major meal. I frequently told others that my body worked like clockwork, and I very much enjoyed my quiet time reading on the 'loo'.

At first, I figured my body was simply feeling the stress from juggling work and being a new dad to young twins. But then I started to feel cramping in my lower back and noticed blood in my stool. My first thought was that it was kidney stones, as this had become somewhat of a regular occurrence over the past five years. I seemed to pass a stone or two every twelve to eighteen months.

In mid-August 2015, a few days after first noticing blood in my stool, I experienced searing pain in my abdomen and checked myself into the emergency room at the hospital. The doctor performed a few routine blood tests and scans. He told me that I didn't have kidney stones and that it was likely colitis, an inflammation of the large intestines. He attributed the blood in my bowels to possible hemorrhoids, since I also had a history of them.

While I was on the antibiotics, the bleeding stopped. However, once I was off them, the pain and bleeding returned. I had already been routinely seeing my GP every two to three weeks for allergy shots (to deal with my severe allergy to pollen), and so at my next appointment, I updated him on my symptoms. He told me in no uncertain terms that what I was experiencing wasn't normal.

My GP scheduled a colonoscopy to make sure things were looking healthy. Unfortunately, due to availability, my procedure would not be until the end of October, but it was only the end of August. My GP wasn't able to reschedule the procedure for any earlier than mid-September, so I resumed life as normal. After the colonoscopy a few weeks later, I was given a sheet of paper with a diagnosis of an ulcer in my colon. Rose and I were relieved. But it was time to clean up my diet.

The following evening my GP called and left me a voice message. He asked how I was feeling, said that he was "sorry" and asked me to call him back. Although I was quite confused by his message, I was already scheduled to see him a few days later for my next allergy shot and decided I would just clarify things with him then.

In retrospect, we should have known. It was unlike him to call. During my appointment he showed me the specialist's report of my colonoscopy and suspected diagnosis: colon cancer.

How was this possible? I had already been diagnosed with an ulcer. I had even nervously and jokingly asked the ER doctor who had given me the ulcer diagnosis back in July, "What is the chance of this being cancer?" To which he had replied, "Based on your age, it's a one in a million chance. For now, you are to finish this course of antibiotics over the next ten days." Now, sitting in my GP's office, I wished I had a recording of that conversation.

My GP told me that we could not move forward with treatment until he received official copies of the scans, verified by at least one other medical professional.

I went home and called Rose with the bad news. She was on her way home from work, and I remember being worried that she would get in an accident. When she got home, she told me to try to look on the brighter side of things. "Lots of people don't die from cancer. It's not necessarily a death sentence." Once the twins were in bed, Rose spent most of that night looking up articles about colon cancer. We decided to keep the news to ourselves until I was officially diagnosed.

Over the course of the next few weeks, we began to see the holes in our medical system and how it was failing us. To receive treatment, I needed my official documentation. To speed up the process, I had to call the specialist's office multiple times. It took me about one week to finally get the paperwork completed so I could be seen by doctors at the BC Cancer Agency.

I was officially diagnosed with cancer on Wednesday, September 21, 2015.

The life I knew fell apart at my feet. I broke the news to my parents over the phone that afternoon. They quickly drove over to be with me, and my mother subsequently called all my siblings and broke the news to them, a few of whom were able to join us. It turned into a crazy night, with all of us sobbing uncontrollably. I knew that Rose was overwhelmed with the chaos. She tried to maintain her composure and tended to the needs of our twins while my parents and I mourned the diagnosis. Our twins had just turned eighteen months old, and all I could think about was how unfair this was.

With Rose's help, I tried to look on the positive side. We told ourselves that as long as we had caught the cancer early, we could overcome this. Rose and I were speculating (and hoping) that I had stage two colon cancer. This would be just a minor hiccup in our journey through life. We had a meeting with our surgical oncologist the next week and were hopeful for a straightforward plan. Rose kept reminding me, "Leave it to God. No amount of worrying will change anything." Of course, that is always easier said than done.

Rose had an open house at work the evening after I told my family. This meant that she had to stay late at work and meet with her students' parents. She had chosen not to tell anyone at work about my cancer diagnosis until she had all the facts and a treatment plan set in motion. So she smiled, meeting with parents and other teachers, and 'did her thing', all with this massive weight on her shoulders. I'm not sure I could've done that.

Since I now had my official diagnosis, I scheduled my medical leave from work to start on Tuesday, October 11, the day after Thanksgiving. This would give me two weeks to tie up any loose ends, ensuring an easy hand-off to my successor. I thought to myself, perhaps this diagnosis was God answering my prayer. I hated my job and was clearly stressed. I needed a break. Maybe this was a part God's plan to grant me rest?

In the days and moments leading up to the meeting with my surgical oncologist, I felt great angst. We kept praying for a silver lining in all this. Someone to confirm that it wasn't too bad. From the moment we met our physician, we knew she had our best interest at heart. She was knowledgeable, efficient and caring. She informed us that I had likely had this tumour for five years, growing undetected despite my seeing a specialist for hemorrhoid removal a few years prior. The cancer itself was now about 9 cm long and located about 10 cm from my anus. Because there were malignant cells in adjacent lymph nodes, I was classified as having stage 3c colon cancer. We were shattered.

A stage three cancer diagnosis also meant that it wasn't a good idea to start treatment with surgery to remove the tumour. Instead, it would be best to first start with radiation to slow down the growth of the tumour and the spread of the cancer. Once the cancer was under control, then the tumour could be surgically removed.

However, there was another complication. Because of the cancer's proximity to the rectum, this sphincter muscle would have to be removed during surgery to ensure that any possible cancer cells in the surrounding regions were eliminated. This would be our best chance at preventing future spreading of the disease. This meant I would need a colostomy, an operation in which my colon would be diverted, bypassing the rectum. I would no longer have bowel movements from my anus, like normal, but rather through a hole in my abdomen. My jaw dropped. I was speechless. This was one more obstacle, one more jab at my pride and yet another means of suffering. There was no way around this.

I said out loud, "You would think, with so many developments in medicine, someone would have invented an artificial rectum." Our doctor laughed and told us to find someone to pitch that idea to. She was truly amazing—an angel, really. She gave us words of encouragement, reminding us, "It's about choosing life, prolonging life. Yes, you will need to make lifestyle changes, but you will be able to spend it with your children. I cannot promise you that this cancer will be gone, but I can tell you that our focus is to prolong your life."

She was right. I wanted to spend as much time with my wife and children as I could. I would adapt. I didn't need to look like a supermodel, I just had to be present and do my part as a husband and father. As I felt a renewed sense of strength and courage, I saw Rose's eyes well up with tears. I knew it was time for me to be the one to put on the brave face.

Our treatment plan was set. We would start with radiation therapy, followed by surgery in February to remove what was left of the cancer and to redirect the colon via a colostomy. If a colostomy meant living to see my children grow up, then so be it. My new mantra became, "I choose life, Lord."

12

Living with Cancer and God at My Side

Perhaps the most frustrating part of my treatment was waiting for my initial radiation session. We felt our life was on hold as we waited in a 'virtual lineup' for a time on the radiation machine. We were somehow not a priority. Rose kept calling the BC Cancer Agency to see why we still had not been given an appointment with the radio-oncologist.

We did finally meet our radio-oncologist about two weeks later, only to have him tell us that it would be yet another two weeks before I could actually receive treatment. This scared me. Even a delay of two weeks would give the cancer more time to grow untreated in my body. Rose began reading medical journals and articles on treatments, prognoses and statistics. We even looked into possible treatment opportunities in the United States. My parents offered to sell their home to support my cancer treatment, should I need it.

Up until this point, my faith had been rocky—I had experienced great highs and low lows. But taking money from my parents felt wrong. Instead, I was going to put my faith in God. He was the author of my life. If I should live, it would be by His hand, not mine or my family's.

My sister and brother-in-law, both faithful Christians, lent me a video called *War Room: Prayer is a Powerful Weapon*. The premise was that through prayer, anything was possible. God hears our cries and will answer us. But since evil can manifest as distractions all around us, why not create a room in our homes designated just for prayer, a room in which to 'take up arms against Satan's ways'? Hence, the movie's title.

War Room inspired Rose to spend more time in prayer. She began to regularly update our electronic prayer request and made our bedroom balcony her 'war room'.

As I saw her trust in God strengthen, I began to wonder where my 'war room' could be. It had to be a place I went to daily, a reminder to commit all my moments to God. I imagined a place that could cover me with His grace. That's when it hit me—water and steam. Those were elements that helped calm me. This is what I could use to help me share my innermost thoughts and listen to Him. My shower—a place I had just to myself, away from distractions, at least twenty minutes every day—would be my 'war room'.

So while Rose used the balcony to surround herself with the natural beauty of the distant mountains, the sounds of birds and the scent of the changing seasons, I washed myself with water, symbolic of the healing waters and spirit of Christ. When days were tough, I found myself taking more than one shower a day.

As I devoted more time to converse with God during my daily steam showers, I felt my conversations with Him deepen. They ranged from me crying out in pain and anger, to smiling in joy as I recalled His blessings and His extreme grace.

It was also at this time that I made a conscious decision, from that day forward, to tell Rose at least once a day the following words: "You are the best thing that happened to me, and the twins are the second."

I had an indescribable bond with my daughter from the day she was born. She ended up saving my life. Isabella saved Daddy!

I'll never forget that night—the night I could have died. We had just celebrated the Thanksgiving weekend. The day after Thanksgiving would be my first official day on medical leave. The twins were sound asleep, and Rose and I were in bed by eleven o'clock.

Around midnight, Isabella woke up screaming and crying. Something wasn't right; it was usually Isaac who woke up. Because I knew Rose had to work the next day, I got out of bed to soothe Bella. As I went to pick her up, I felt warm liquid running down my leg. I quickly called Rose to hold Bella while I went to see what was happening. To my horror, there was a steady flow of blood coming from my rectum.

I rushed into the bathtub. It wasn't just blood, it was congealed. I was hemorrhaging. I had seen this before—only last time it had been happening to Rose, after her delivery of the twins. Now it was my turn. I hated the sight of blood in general, but now I was scared. It was my own! Rose quickly called 911. She then called her sister to come spend the night with the twins so she could be by my side at the hospital.

We were truly thankful and blessed that only Bella had woken up that night. Isaac continued to sleep peacefully. The ambulance arrived quickly, as did my sister-in-law. I somehow managed to get downstairs before feeling light-headed from all the blood loss. I don't remember much of what happened after the ambulance arrived. The following is Rose's account:

> Wilson's situation was quite serious and scary. The amount of blood loss reminded me of my own hemorrhage one and a half years earlier. The blood clots, coagulated chunks of blood, would not stop flowing.
>
> Once we knew the ambulance was on its way, Wilson insisted on meeting the paramedics on the main floor. While I had wanted him to remain upstairs, he was adamant. He told me he didn't want anyone coming upstairs, and he felt he was strong enough to walk. Once on the main floor, Wilson noticed that he had left trail of blood behind him. Because he is Wilson, he then attempted to clean up after himself, not only because he didn't want to burden me with another task, but because he wanted to make sure he didn't stain our floors! I told him to stop being ridiculous and that I would deal with the mess later.
>
> The ambulance and my sister arrived at the same time. I quickly handed Bella to my sister and asked her to wait in the family room while I spoke to the paramedics.
>
> Once Wilson was in the ambulance, I told my sister that I would be back in the morning to attend to the twins. When I arrived at Vancouver General Hospital's ER, the nurses were collecting and weighing Wilson's blood output, but there was too much. They moved him to a portable toilet, but by then Wilson was too weak to even sit up for more than a few moments.
>
> Even though they had moved us to a triage unit, the other two individuals in the room with us were also in quite a serious

condition. One was a burn victim and the other was a 'John Doe' flown in from the Interior. Someone had found him in the woods, thinking he was dead. He had suffered a severe blow to his spine and would likely become a quadriplegic.

While the nurses and doctors were tending to and assessing the other two cases, I was actively involved in disposing of the coagulated blood exiting Wilson's body. The ward was short-staffed, and it was clear that my presence in the ER was necessary, as I was literally collecting and disposing of excess blood clots in a dustpan every few minutes. With this rate of blood loss, the doctors set him up for a blood transfusion.

Wilson had started bleeding shortly before midnight. It was now four o'clock. The doctors told me that if there was no sign of the hemorrhage slowing down in the next few hours, they would cancel the blood transfusion as it would have been point-less; any new blood entering his body would be shortly exiting it. I was a nervous wreck. I began to panic. My life was unravelling before my very eyes. There was a good chance that Wilson was going to die.

I remember praying to God, asking for more time. I was not ready to lose the love of my life ... not yet.

I called in sick to work. By the time I was ready to leave the hospital to check up on the twins and relieve my sister at seven o'clock, Wilson's condition seemed to have stabilized. The ER doctor told me that because Wilson had cancer, we had to wait for an oncologist to see him before anything further could be done. Nothing was clear-cut.

When I stepped into our house, I was met by Wilson's mom. His parents were distraught. It was supposed to be a normal babysitting day for them. They knew something was wrong as soon as they saw my sister's car parked in front of our house. I explained Wilson's situation to them. I told them I was home to check on the twins and that I needed to be back at the hospital as soon as possible. When I returned to VGH around 9:30 a.m., Wilson had just received six units of trans-fused blood.

In my mind, all I could ask was, "Lord, what is happening?"

Besides immediate family members and doctors, I remember talking to two people that day—my union rep and Wilson's best friend. Both told me that I had to keep it together—the twins needed me. That became my mantra. I knew God had a plan.

I prayed.

I begged.

I cried.

Over the course of the next twelve hours, we learned that the hemorrhage was most likely caused by a burst blood vessel, one that had been feeding the tumour. Because surgery to remove the tumour was scheduled for post radiation, the ER doctors could not go in and deal directly with the infected area. Wilson's treatment protocol had to first be reviewed by the oncology team.

Radiation treatment before tumour removal could potentially kill any cancer cells migrating out of the initial site, thereby minimizing the spread of cancer to other regions in his body. It was recommended that this section of the colon be as "undisturbed as possible"—meaning no feces could pass through. In short, Wilson needed a colostomy, stat! What we had discussed with the surgical oncologist was coming to fruition on a much faster timeline than we had expected.

Wilson was so brave! He said, "I choose life. It's just a bag. I will adjust. I want to be here to see the twins grow up." I felt so proud that this was the man I married.

Although our surgical oncologist was out of town, God planned for there to be another reliable and experienced surgeon available to lead the surgery. It was a success! But, as brave as Wilson was, he was disheartened by and very self-conscious of his new body. I did what I could to be the best support for him.

Anyone who really knows me knows that my mind works sequentially and logically. My mind was on autopilot wondering what the next step would be and then how to get there in the most efficient time frame. I couldn't help but feel like we were constantly behind the eight ball. If we could just get ahead, we might have a chance to beat this cancer.

Wilson's first radiation treatment was to start in the next few days. I was already disheartened that radiation treatment hadn't started before this hemorrhaging fiasco, and I definitely didn't want any further delays, so I followed up with our radio-oncologist. To my shock, he had no idea that Wilson was in the hospital, much less now with a colostomy! I gave him a detailed account of Wilson's new physiology. With the new changes in his body, Wilson would now require a new radiation protocol. This meant another two- to three-week delay before radiation could actually begin.

While Rose was trying to get all of my doctors on the same page, I had a chance to really rest. During my two-week stay in the hospital, I felt great love. I was visited by many friends. I was amazed that, even in this craziness, Rose was still able to keep things in perspective. She travelled back and forth between the hospital and home to ensure the twins didn't feel abandoned.

Rose also inadvertently became a counsellor for my parents. Because her parents were out of town while I was in the hospital, my parents were over every day to help us with the twins. Rose told me my father literally shut down for three days. He just sat in our family room, staring into space, while my mother burned incense, blared a pre-recorded Buddhist chant on the main floor and prayed repeatedly.

I'm sure it was a déjà vu moment for my mother, as this was something she had already done for me once before, back in Thailand after my cranial surgery. I know she was asking Buddha and our ancestors for help to heal me. Although Rose was clearly agitated by their religious acts of desperation, she did her best to understand and relate to my parents.

Once I was discharged from the hospital, I knew Rose was walking a fine line between sanity and madness. She returned to work full-time shortly after I settled back at home but planned to take a longer leave of absence in February to care for me after my tumor removal surgery. Between work and home, Rose was truly hanging on by a thread. She was there every step of the way to support me, and it was easier to walk this path knowing I wasn't alone. Rose also became my stoma care aid. Together, we cared for and changed my ostomy bags. She read up on literature so I could eat foods that would support my digestive health and regulate the consistency of my bowel movements.

Although Rose knew how ugly I felt because of my stoma, she regularly reminded me that she loved me regardless of how I looked. I understood that I was still the same person—bag or no bag—but I was having a hard time accepting my new lifestyle. I couldn't help but feel self-conscious. Even if others couldn't tell I had an ostomy bag, I knew

I had one. I loved swimming and massages from an RMT (registered massage therapist), but now there was no way I was going to let someone else see or touch me with this ugly thing on my body. However, I knew I had to be around to watch and be a part of our twins' lives. They were so precious. It would be very selfish of me to leave Rose to raise them on her own. She needed me.

Although I had a colostomy to bypass the last segment of my colon and rectum, those muscles were still active. Peristalsis, an involuntary wave-like motion that moves food and liquid through the esophagus and intestines, was still happening, even though no digested food was present. As a result, my body was still producing gastric juices and pushing mucus, our body's natural lubricant, out through my rectum. I often complained to Rose about the constant "leakage." Fortunately, this would end once I received my surgery in the next few months. In the interim, I began wearing Rose's sanitary napkins. It became an inside joke between us that I now knew how it felt to have a period.

I also complained about the inconvenience of not being able to control my bowel movements and the physical presence of ostomy bags. How could I go back to work like this? I hate admitting this, but I suffered from OCD. I developed a habit of constantly touching and rubbing my stoma. Once I had a bowel movement, I had to empty and rinse my bag right away because I was self-conscious about constantly smelling like fecal matter.

Rose tried to encourage me and keep my spirits up. She said that we could have a 'new normal', one where I could still do the things I enjoyed like swimming and going to work. She reminded me that when things calmed down and we had the cancer under control, we could try irrigation, a process shared with us by our ostomy nurse. This hour-long process would allow me to better control my bowel movements so that I would not have to worry about emptying my ostomy bag. This method required using water to flush and empty my colon at a scheduled time, mainly in the comfort of my own home. The water flushed into my colon would stimulate my colon to empty. Even though Rose was excited to share this process with me, I was rather hesitant as I'm not into trying new things. What if it didn't work for me?

As I settled into the new normal, radiation was added to my schedule. The first month of treatment was okay, but starting in November, my anal region became very tender and eventually it was unbearably painful. I became irritable despite being on a pretty high dose of pain medications.

111

With Rose at work, I found myself talking to God more and more. I asked Him to help ease the pain. I began watching movies based on the Bible and started listening to sermons online.

Since Rose was working, she couldn't come to every appointment with me. She told me to bring up my pain with the radiologist or my family doctor, but I didn't. A part of me felt that things were complicated enough. I figured the issue would resolve itself, or if it were really that bad, someone would take notice. (It's like asking for directions to go somewhere. I just don't like asking. That's why I generally had Rose do the asking.)

Maybe it was also my way of having Rose show me that I was still important and loved. By December, she had had enough of my complaining and took matters into her own hands. She called our radio-oncologist directly and told him about my pain, then asked if a suppository could be prescribed to help. He agreed it could and quickly had a prescription made out so that we could pick up the medication.

I wondered in awe about Rose's ability to come up with pragmatic solutions. When asked, she would tell me to thank the Lord for His wisdom. "I just listen," she said. I am thankful that Rose picks up on His intentions. The suppositories provided instant relief, and once the suppositories resolved my localized pain, I immediately began weaning myself off oxycodone to ensure I didn't begin to overly rely on it, perhaps even permanently.

Beginning January 2016, I was finally comfortable with my stoma. I had settled into my new routine, especially since my radiation treatments were finally over. According to the surgical oncologist's original plan, I was to go in for surgery the following month. However, after careful discussion with the team, it was determined that before surgery, it would be best that I start my first round of chemotherapy using FOLFOX, containing Folinic Acid (FOL), Fluorouracil (F) and Oxaliplatin (OX). My surgery was postponed once again, this time to May.

Rose and I were at the mercy of the decisions of these doctors. With the updated protocol for treatment, Rose still wanted to take her leave mid-February to spend more time with me. She said it was important that she be at all my appointments. She didn't want to just be my moral support, but more importantly she wanted to be present at my appointments to actively ask clarifying questions about my treatment.

It was soon recommended that I have a PowerPort installed to receive chemotherapy. A PowerPort is an implant placed just under the surface of the skin that allows quick access to the venous system for easy infusion of medications and for drawing blood for testing. Having this port would ensure I would always have access to chemo, and I wouldn't have to wait for a chair to be available.

My chemotherapy treatment would start at the end of January. Since I was on medical leave, I needed to keep myself busy while Rose was still at work and the twins were being taken care of by our parents. I decided to start being more physically active, so I began to walk every day—sometimes for up to three hours. I would often walk myself to different casinos, movie theatres and lunch destinations. Because I had lost a significant amount of weight, many of my other health issues began to disappear. I no longer needed cholesterol or diabetes pills, and even my sleep apnea lessened.

During my daily walks, I listened to music. Slowly, my music turned to the audio Bible and then to church sermons online. I could not help but feel an innate desire to change. I soon went from walking to casinos to volunteering my time at Union Gospel Mission. When chemotherapy started, I even walked an hour to the Cancer Agency for my treatments.

While I was extremely grateful that I no longer experienced pain in my rectal region and that I had successfully weaned myself off of my pain medication, I was prescribed a whole different set of drugs pre- and post-chemo. Although I hated injecting my body with these toxins, I had minimal side effects. I didn't lose much hair, but I did feel mildly nauseated a few days before and after each treatment.

I had great friends—another one of God's provisions. To help me pass the time while the chemo medication was infused into my body, a process that took at least two hours, different sets of friends would come by and keep me company. What I dreaded the most about chemo days was carrying a "slow-dispensing chemo bottle" for another day after leaving the Cancer Agency.

The chemo rendered me weaker than usual, and my family was careful to ensure that only healthy people entered our home because of my compromised immune system. To support Rose, I took on the task of putting the twins to bed each night. Rose would shower them and read them at least one book and a Bible story before I took over. The twins would be in their separate beds with me lying on a mattress on the floor between them. I would tell them I loved them, sing and pray with them and play music softly in the background as I held their little hands to help settle them to sleep. This time spent waiting for them to sleep, anywhere from fifteen to forty minutes, eventually morphed into my own time of self-reflection.

Rose had brought up the question of baptism at our recent meeting with our life group. She had put me on the spot and asked why I didn't want to be baptized. I told her that I didn't feel the need, for if God truly knew my heart, He would see that I believed. Rose wasn't buying it, but she knew further probing wouldn't change my decision. It had to come from me.

It was during these quiet moments lying with my children while they fell asleep that I could truly see myself 'naked' before God. This was when it all struck me—hard. I had had a tough life. Nothing had come easily. I had made it out of Cambodia during the height of the Khmer Rouge, survived the civil war in Vietnam and even my fall while in a refugee camp in Thailand. But I knew now that my survival was not the result of my own actions alone. I could now confidently say that the Lord had been with me every step of the way.

God had been performing miracles in front of my eyes—for me. Why had it taken me so long to see Him? I was now able to clearly see that it was God's hand that moved our sinking boat to the shores of Thailand. It was God's hand that ensured a ready and willing brain surgeon was there to perform the life-saving surgery after my fall. It was Jesus who carried me on His back to recovery.

Miracle upon miracle…

As a ten-year-old, while out for a bike ride, I had managed to slide under a large, oncoming cargo truck without injury, except for a few scratches on my knee. I had been saved by the small metal frame of my bike. Then, as an adult, I narrowly avoided losing my life while driving home from a work trip in icy conditions along the Coquihalla Highway. Six months after surrendering my desire for children to God, it was Jesus who sent me a message to look to Thailand. God performed miracle upon miracle to prove His love for me.

In looking back, I know now that I had been blinded by Satan's plan of deception. Satan had planted seeds of doubt, and I hadn't uprooted them. Instead, I had let those bad seeds stay, and those seeds had taken root. Soon those roots of doubt had become vines of doubt—snuffing out the significance of every miracle God had performed.

I was overwhelmed by a strong sense of shame. How could I have denied His very existence for so long? I was filled with emotion and a

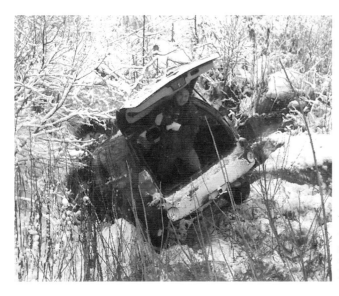

Wilson retrieving the company GPS, after his accident on the Coquihalla Highway

sense of conviction. From this day forward, I would let God's love supersede my seeds of doubt. My new mantra was "No more to Lucifer!"

Funny enough, in a conversation at my place a few weeks later, my brother-in-law told me he was going to be baptized in his home, along with his two boys, in about a month's time. He went on to ask me if I wanted to join them. I felt overcome with a sense of peace, and I said, "Yes!"

I felt ready to commit my life fully to God. I was going to be baptized with family members in my sister's home. Rose walked in and overheard parts of our conversation. She was ecstatic! It was clear to her that God was using my brother-in-law to draw me home. Here is an excerpt from my testimony:

> In the last few months, I have been brought to my knees from pain, and yet despite all the poor decisions I have made to dishonour God, Jesus still sent relief. Today, February 6, 2016, although I am marred with the battle scars of cancer—a cancer that has now spread to my liver—today, I declare, "No more!" I say "No more" to Lucifer! Because when I am baptized in the blood of Jesus, it will wash away my sin and along with it, the seed, the root and the vines of doubt. I rise from this knowing that the Lord has walked with me all along the way.

I continued with the chemo treatment until mid-April. Based on my recent blood test and scans, it was apparent that the chemo had not been as effective as we had hoped. Unfortunately, the cancer was still spreading. Despite this sad news, I was excited that my chemo treatment was finished so that this tumour could finally be removed from my body. Once the tumour was removed, tissue samples could be sent for POG (personalized oncogenetics) testing. Some patients have been able to receive more targeted and effective treatments based on the information from the tissue samples. We were hopeful that our doctors could learn more information that would benefit our battle.

My original surgery date was scheduled for May 24, 2016, but our surgical oncologist's mother suddenly passed away, and our doctor had to fly back to Germany for two weeks. My surgery date was pushed back to June 8, 2016.

Due to the postponement of my surgery, I ended up missing a family reunion on Quadra Island. My mom stayed behind to be with me so Rose could take the twins. Although I was disappointed, there was a silver lining. I was able to spend quality time with my mom.

The surgery to remove the tumour went well. I had two surgeons working on me—one to remove the large tumour in my colon and another to remove the new, smaller tumours in my liver. The surgery was quite invasive, and I had a massive scar down the centre of my chest. Once I was discharged from the hospital, I required daily visits from home care nurses to monitor my incisions and stitches.

The recovery process was hard. I had stitches and swelling, the result of having had my chest and abdominal cavity opened and my anal region sewn shut. I was in so much pain afterward that I spent most of my time lying in bed, on pain medication. I had no appetite.

There were moments when I just wanted it all to end. The pain was intense. I could barely move. I couldn't sleep. It was hard to lie in any one position. In fact, any movement led to great discomfort, even agony. A few times a day, I forced myself out of bed to sit on a special air cushion, called the ROHO cushion. Although a nurse came to change my dressings once a day, I needed more help than that. Rose took on the additional responsibility of changing my dressings every three to four hours.

My post-op visit with the surgical oncologist, two weeks after my surgery, was disheartening. My pathology report indicated that the cancer was back. It had metastasized to other parts of my body before we had a chance to remove the original tumour. Furthermore, my chemotherapy treatment of FOLFOX was having little to no effect on slowing down the cancer.

I now had stage four colon cancer. Despite being hit with the disappointing news, we were still hopeful that the next round of chemo would be more effective.

By mid-August, my scans showed that I had a new lesion on my liver and a possible tumour behind my stoma. There were also cancerous cells in the lymph nodes in my abdomen, side and chest. Furthermore, one of my surgical wounds was still not fully healed. Starting chemo now would only further slow my healing process and allow opportunities for complications with infections. However, given the aggressive nature of my cancer, doctors recommended that I take the risk and start my last round of chemo, FOLFIRI with bevacizumab, at the beginning of September.

From his conversations with another chemotherapist, my oncologist informed us that while FOLFOX had shown to be effective in 65 percent of the population, the efficacy of FOLFIRI was only 50 percent. The eradication of my cancer was unlikely. The chemotherapy would instead be used to keep the cancer under control, in an effort to prolong my life.

We had to change our mindset. We would now need to think of cancer as an inconvenience like diabetes, and not necessarily a death sentence. With this new mindset, Rose planned to return to work full-time, and I thought about what life would look like for me as I lived harmoniously with cancer. I actually felt stronger as I weaned myself off my pain medications. I even started to feel semi-normal.

Although I knew I needed the chemotherapy, I really dreaded the process. I hated the way the pre- and post-chemo drugs made me feel, and I detested the stench of the Cancer Agency. To minimize my trips to the Agency, Rose even learned how to remove my slow-release diffusion bottle at home.

After months of waiting, our POG results came in, and unfortunately they were inconclusive. We had hoped that I had a cancer that could be fought using immunotherapy. This news made me feel defeated and depressed.

With Rose now back at work full-time, I spent most of my days on my own. During this time, everyone and their dog had an opinion about what I should and shouldn't eat. Since my cancer diagnosis, Rose had limited my beef intake to once a month. My primary diet was smoothies, fish and chicken. But I didn't have just any run-of-the-mill smoothies, mine were pretty special. And by that, I mean pretty nasty. Rose read up on all things 'anti-cancerous' and loaded up my smoothies with fresh beets, celery root, cumin, oregano, fresh turmeric and aloe vera, home-made fermented black garlic, cayenne and glutamine powder. This made for an intensely thick shake! I called it my poison. I also took daily reishi mushroom pills, and my mother would make me braised sea cucumber at least once a week. At one point, I was even drinking dandelion tea!

During one of my daily walks after consuming my anti-cancer shake, I was overwhelmed with fear. For the first time in my life, I recognized how precious time was and that there was no way I could control the outcome of my life.

I later confessed to Rose that I was feeling depressed and suicidal. I was losing my drive to live. I was coming to terms with the fact that I was dying. I started to look into the process of transferring assets into her name and contacting people to help Rose claim my life insurance when I passed away. I needed to ensure she wasn't left with a big burden. We even bought into a death insurance plan that would help walk us through details to plan my funeral.

For the first time in many years, I began to withdraw and distance myself from the ones who loved me most. Rose quickly noticed the change and suggested I go for counselling. She also wondered if I was suffering as a result of weaning myself off painkillers, a narcotic called OxyNEO. I told her I didn't want to talk to a counsellor and asked, "How are they going to help me? I don't want to talk to anybody. What are they going to tell me that I don't already know?"

To which Rose said, "Then interact with others by volunteering somewhere locally. You told me you wanted to give back to the community. Here is your chance." So I did. I had often told Rose that I wanted to sleep on the streets of Chinatown for a few nights to experience what it would be like to be homeless. I wanted to get to know people who felt abandoned. Thus, it made sense that I begin volunteering downtown at Union Gospel Mission, or UGM. I made an instant connection with the volunteer director when I interviewed for the position.

My first shift was in mid-September 2016. I was to stock items for sale in the back room of the thrift store to minimize contact with others and lessen my chance of contracting an infection since I was on chemo. But I was bored without anyone to interact with, so I requested a new position. I was moved to an office setting, which I much preferred. It actually felt like I was back at work.

Around this time, Rose and I also spoke to a member of our extended family, a professional financial advisor, about our financial situation and what our plan would look like when I passed away. I had to ensure that Rose and the twins would be okay financially. I told Rose that, should the need arise, she had to sell our home. I advised her, "Don't keep this house for me!"

However, it was the other things we addressed during this financial talk that struck us most. I always knew I wanted to be cremated and have my ashes scattered in the ocean, especially since I loved swimming and being near the water. But it was when we were asked to think about how Rose could 'keep me alive' for the twins in their milestone moments like their first day of kindergarten, their first dates, their graduation from high school and their weddings that I felt daggers drive deep into my heart.

Oh, how I wanted to be there to have a father–daughter dance with Bella and to give her away to her future husband at her wedding! When it was suggested that a cremation urn be present, or a scattering of my ashes could be saved for those occasions, I nodded my head and wept. That night, Rose looked into purchasing cremation necklaces for the twins when I died, so that a part of me could be physically present with them.

Although I was happy that my second round of chemo was over in mid-November, there would be no official treatment protocol after this stage—we were running out of options. Rose and I dreaded our last appointment with the chemotherapist. Although we braced ourselves for sad news, we still hoped for a light at the end of this tunnel.

We knew time was something we didn't have. Just six months before, Rose had asked our surgical oncologist how long I would have once we exhausted our prescribed treatment protocol. At the time, she had said I'd have about two more years. And so Rose had realistically braced herself for at least two more years together. But in my mind, I wanted ten. Just ten years, Lord. I wanted a chance to see my twins grow up. To have them remember me. Thus, when on Friday, December 2, 2016, our chemo-oncologist told us that this was potentially my last Christmas, our hearts sank.

This was a day to remember. It was a signal that my journey on Earth was about to end. Rose choked up, unable to stop the steady stream of tears from rolling down her face, and neither could I. It took us a good two weeks to get out from under a thick cloud of darkness.

Over the prior months, both Rose and I had been reading about the advancements in cancer treatment resulting from immunotherapy. Instead of injecting a toxin into your body (chemotherapy) that eliminates both good and bad cells, immunotherapy uses your body's own immune system to fight the cancer. One reason that cancer can remain undetected in our bodies for so long is that our immune system doesn't recognize cancer cells as 'foreign' cells. But in the case of immunotherapy, our system is stimulated to attack these cancer cells.

When we asked our chemotherapist about this, he told us that only a limited number of clinical trials were currently available for colon cancer patients. There just wasn't as much public outpouring of funds going toward research for colorectal cancer compared to breast or lung cancer. Hence, there hadn't been as many advancements in treatment.

In terms of trying experimental options and participating in clinical trials, we had to wait for one to become available and then to qualify for it. At that point, there was only one proven effective immunotherapy option available to colon cancer patients, but I didn't qualify for it because I did not have the mutant form of the KRAS gene that was required for the therapy to be effective.

There was one final option—an immunotherapy pilot beginning at the end January 2017. However, this was a brand new trial, where one group would receive a placebo treatment while the other would get the experimental drug. Drug recipient patients would be chosen based on a lottery system. In the original proposal, the trial was a 'double blind' set-up, meaning patients would not know if they were getting a bag of saline or one with the trial drug infused with saline. It was deemed that a patient's not knowing infringed on their rights, and thus, the trial did not pass the medical board of ethics. Two months later, the trial parameters were changed so that patients would be told at the beginning of the trial if they were receiving treatment or not.

I felt pressured to do something other than just sit around waiting two months for this new immunology trial. There was yet another drug trial that I could participate in, which involved the use of blood pressure pills to control cancer cell growth. I was all in, but Rose was not. In her pragmatism, she asked what the side effects would be. Most patients in the trial reported developing sores on the palms of their hands and soles of their feet. Rose paused before asking, "How much longer do the patients actually live?"

The doctor's response was "six weeks." Rose was exasperated, "What? Six weeks? That's it? It wouldn't be an additional six weeks of quality life if you are dealing with sores so bad that you can't even walk!"

But I was insistent on participating in the trial. It was my decision, my body. I wanted to live. Maybe I would be lucky and not have any side effects.

To qualify for the trial, I had to have normal blood pressure. I knew this wouldn't be a problem since my blood pressure had stabilized to normal over the last two years as I had lost weight from the cancer and treatment. I was slated to start the trial in mid-December 2016, but when I went in for my screening, my blood pressure was suddenly all over the place! The nurse told me I could come back and see her the next day to retest my blood pressure. I went home devastated.

When I told Rose about the situation, she said, "I bet it's God telling you this drug trial is not for you. The reward of a possible six weeks of life is not worth enduring sores on your hands and feet in addition to the pain you already have. God's stopping you because you are now just grasping at anything. We need to wait for that immunotherapy drug trial. We can pray that you will be one of the lucky ones that gets the medication."

Rose knew the importance and power of prayer. According to 1 John 5:14–15, "This is the confidence that we have toward him, that if we ask anything according to his will, he hears us. And if we know that he hears us in whatever we ask, we know that we have the requests that we have asked of him." So instead of calling people individually to update family and friends on Wilson's progress, Rose created an email prayer chain that she diligently updated and shared via email. We prayed for strength, wisdom, courage and above all else—miraculous healing. We had friends regularly visiting us to share their love and support.

Before the end of the year, and just a few weeks prior to the immunotherapy trial, I began to experience pain in my abdomen again. It was also around this time that we noticed some bumps around my stoma. Rose instructed me to ask my stoma nurse about them at my next visit. When I did, the nurse thought they might simply be skin irritation from the adhesive on the ostomy bags, so we tried using different ointments and brands to see if this resolved the issue.

Recent scans also showed that the cancer was spreading. It was now pushing against my ureters, and I would eventually need a stent surgically placed to ensure these tubes didn't collapse. A procedure called a nephrostomy was now on the horizon. We were pencilled in for early February 2017.

Over the next few weeks, I spun myself into another depression. I knew I was dying, but I didn't want to let Rose down. I had to live for her and the twins. I was in so much physical pain. I was tired of feeling sick and weak. I hated not being able to help Rose with the twins and not having the energy to go out. I hated the fact that I had no control and that there was no solution to kick this cancer. I couldn't sleep. I kept replaying how I could have changed the outcome of my life. To distract my mind from suicidal thoughts, I watched TV. Rose did her best to be with me, and when she couldn't 'get to me', she arranged for friends to be around me.

With Christmas and my forty-third birthday fast approaching, my sister-in-law arranged a small birthday dinner at an expensive steakhouse restaurant with my closest friends and family members. According to my chemo-oncologist, this would likely be my last birthday celebration and steak dinner. As a I blew out the candle on my slice of cake, I secretly wished for more time.

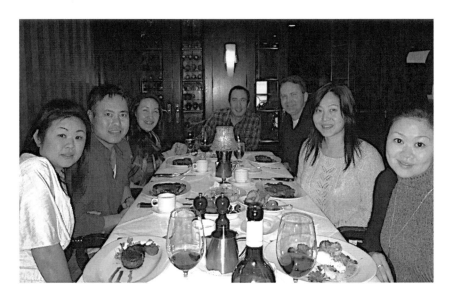

From left to right: Rose, Wilson, friends and family members

13

Final Days

Because I desperately wanted to live, and because I had already tried everything medically available to me, a close friend of ours suggested spiritual healing. Since this was the only option left on the table, I thought, "Why not?" I wasn't sure what to expect, but I was secretly hoping for something new and profound.

A week later, during a healing session in my dining room, the prayer healer asked me, "Wilson, what do you see?"

My eyes were closed, and my body was relaxed. As I sat on my dining chair, I told him emphatically, "I see nothing…"

He asked me to quiet my mind. "Don't try to analyze what you see."

After a minute or two, I began to see something formulate. But it didn't make any sense. "I see a colourful parrot…"

The healer continued, "Do you see anything else?"

I tried to calm my mind as I focused on the colours of the parrot. "I see the cross…"

"Do you see anything else?"

I continued to focus on this white cross, but I didn't see anything else. Justin, our spiritual healer, said, "Wilson, God wants you to take that cross and put it on."

I wasn't sure what Justin meant. "How do I do that?"

I felt Justin take my hands in his. Together we reached out and grabbed the cross and pushed it into my chest. Justin asked, "Wilson, how do you feel?"

I felt a warmth emanating from my chest, and I had a tingly sensation move throughout my body. The unrelenting pain in my body subsided. I yelled, "Wow! The pain is almost gone! Thank you, Jesus!"

After our healing session, Justin looked up what it meant to envision a parrot. One website mentioned that a parrot appears to you when you need a new perspective on your future and encourages you to achieve new goals with ease and confidence. A second website noted that the parrot is a happy expression of all the good things around you and a reminder to never take these things for granted. It reminds us to focus on love and friendship.

Although these meanings made sense, I was still a little disappointed. Although I felt physically better, I had wanted a definitive sign from God that I would kick this cancer.

Over the course of the next few days, Rose commented that I seemed more energetic and spiritually alert. I wasn't as focused on my physical pain; I seemed more at ease and less irritated. She immediately began looking for other healing rooms around the city.

Soon after, on December 29, 2016, God led us to an open prayer session at The Healing Room in Chinatown. We arrived early and were invited to take part in their morning circle. One of the men, a tall, lanky older gentleman, ironically named Tiny, slowly walked around the room, spending a few minutes with each of the attendees, proclaiming a special message to us from God. Rose recognized how special this opportunity was and quickly whipped out her phone to record the message he had for us.

Bear in mind that this was the first time we had met each other; Tiny knew nothing about us except that I had cancer. When it was my turn, Tiny asked me to stand up. This was already strange as he had not asked anyone else to stand. Tiny said:

> The Lord is asking you to stand up for Jesus. You have been hesitant with the Lord, but you have had the best walk ever. Stand up for Him. Don't hold back. Your heart will change the hearts of others. I can see that you have released your life to the Lord. Our kingdom needs more men, and I can see Jesus raising up men to draw others home, too. People will see a change in you

and ask themselves, "Who is this guy?" I can see the Holy Spirit working through you to move others to stand up for Jesus. Lord, help Wilson bring a load of men to Christ.

In that moment, I knew Tiny was right. I had been jumping on and off the Christian bandwagon for years, always wanting to be a faithful soldier for Christ but never feeling like I was good enough. But here God was reminding me that I had to stand up for Him. He was counting on me. My life had a purpose.

As Tiny began to deliver a message to the person sitting next to me, my mind began spinning, wondering how I could fulfill God's task. Shortly after this morning circle, the attendees were divided in two, and I was invited to enter a separate room to receive prayer alongside one of the groups. I shared with them that I had cancer and that I wished for physical and spiritual healing. I told them that I felt I may have brought this illness upon myself, saying, "I believe I made a deal with the Devil. In my frustration and sadness, I told him I'd be willing to shorten my life to have kids."

As tears welled in my eyes, I continued, "I have no regrets. My children are worth it. I just never imagined myself dying so soon. I want more time..."

One of the team members led me in a prayer to spiritually 'unbind' myself from this contract I had signed with the Devil. Shortly afterward, Rose was invited into the room so we could all receive another round of prayers together.

We both left The Healing Room spiritually refreshed. On our way home, I told Rose that I wanted to start a new chapter in my life. I wanted to live to honour God. I wanted to minister to families struck by cancer. I could tell Rose was excited. She immediately supported my decision and told me that she could reduce her hours at work to support me in my ministry.

Christmas came and went like in previous years, but it felt different. It was potentially my last one. We spent a quiet night at home on New Year's Eve, and because our kids hadn't yet mastered sleeping through the night, Rose and I took turns checking on them, providing comfort when they woke up screaming from night terrors. I wanted them to know I was close by. But on this last night of 2016, I found that I was in constant pain and easily irritated. And so, as the new year began, Rose took that first evening shift.

With the coming of the new year, it felt as if there was a sudden and definite change in my physical and mental state. Over the next few weeks, Rose would often ask me to accompany her on her walks with the twins: "How about a short walk to Trout Lake? The lake actually froze over this year! If not that, how about the mall? The twins would really enjoy an outing…" Of course, it wasn't really for the twins. Rose wanted to get me out the house, out of the chair in the family room.

After much prompting, I finally agreed. We managed to make it to the mall. I told myself to keep it together for my kids. We boarded the parent-and-tot mini train ride at the mall, and I lasted all of five minutes before I said, "Rose, I'm done. I'm in too much pain. My stomach hurts."

I could see the disappointment in her eyes, but I just couldn't do it. Since my birthday dinner, despite taking pain medication, I was in a state of chronic pain. It affected my ability to sleep at night, so I eventually opted to sit and try to sleep on the recliner in front of the TV so Rose could get some quality rest.

Soon my condition worsened to the point where I couldn't eat or drink without serious abdominal cramping. I couldn't help but feel the end was near. I wanted to stay with Rose and the twins…as long as I could.

14

Wilson's Legacy
(written by Rose, with Wilson's reflections in italics)

I admitted Wilson to Emergency at VGH on January 31, 2017. Doctors quickly discovered that it was an intestinal blockage that had been causing Wilson's pain. It was during the next eight weeks that we both witnessed the amazing work of God all around us.

In facing all the downward turns and obstacles, Wilson continued to show great courage, stamina and perseverance. During my evening visits to the hospital, Wilson and I would walk around the unit and sit in the patient lounge overlooking the stunning Vancouver landscape—views of the harbour and majestic mountains. We sat quietly holding hands, wondering when this chapter would end and what would come next. Wilson would remind me how much he loved me and the twins, and how sorry he was to be leaving us.

One of these nights, shortly before falling asleep, Wilson told me that I had to go on living my life: "Your ties to me are done. If you meet someone, don't hold back. I give you my blessing." I remember telling him to not be silly and that things would be okay.

During Wilson's stay in the hospital, we had many friends offer and say healing prayers over us. Wilson even went out on a day pass to attend a special service at Bethel Church.

It was so weird. I was in so much pain. The pain medication seemed to be wearing off. I wanted to stay for the service. But I couldn't. I just remember these people surrounding my wheelchair, praying over me.... Then I blacked out. I could sense that someone was screaming in the background. I felt a strong force of light come over me. I felt instantly filled with love and power. I knew this feeling. There was no doubt in my mind that this was Jesus. I gave in to the light. The next thing I knew, I was alert. I felt completely at ease and my pain was gone! As I looked around and saw my wife and parents, I felt a sense of gratitude. One of the prayer team members asked me how I felt. I said, "Amazing! I want to stand up and walk."

I still pinch myself, a reminder that this really happened. "Stand up. Stand up for Jesus." Those were the words that came to mind. A reminder of what Tiny had said only a little over a month prior. God had orchestrated this event at Bethel Church so well. Even Wilson's parents—non-believers—were witnesses. Wilson not only felt God's power, but more importantly recognized the gift the Lord had given him. And all the while surrounded by friends and family.

I was comforted knowing with absolute certainty that Heaven existed and that Wilson and I would be together again at some point in the future. One morning, not long after our time at Bethel Church, God whispered to me, "Rose, I have raised you and prepared you for such a time as this."

I was going in for a scope of my colon. I braced myself for bad news. Over the last few weeks, things had been going from bad to worse. But maybe, just this time, Rose would tell me something different...

I couldn't help but feel blessed that God had paired me with Rose. She was so strong. She was my crutch. Yet, I was so tired. I was beginning to feel selfish as I wanted to go home to God. I didn't want to live like this anymore. Cancer was winning the battle over my physical body.

On this same day, I would experience one of the hardest moments of my life. I had to tell the one I loved that he was going to die. That he wouldn't be coming home to be with me and the twins.

Rose and I had been together for so long that I knew what she would say before words left her mouth. So when she entered the room with tears welling in her eyes, I knew my time was coming to an end. I reached out for her hand. As we silently took a good long look at each other, time seemed to stand still.

I had been running a race that I knew I couldn't win, but up until this very moment, I had glimmers of hope that it was still possible. I wanted a miracle for Wilson. He had been so brave throughout the last year and half. It was in this moment that he began to cry.

Rose, I'm sorry. I can't raise the twins with you, and I can't grow old with you. I want to go home for one last time. I want a farewell party. I want a chance to see and thank all my friends. Rose, I want you to order some Vietnamese subs for the guests. I can be seated in the living room. Then after the party, I want to come back to the hospital and spend some time with my siblings, parents, you and the twins before falling asleep to go home with Jesus.

I quickly began to plan for his special party with our palliative care doctor. Later that evening, one of my sisters-in-law texted me and told us that her pastor wanted to pray with us over the phone. After we hung up, Wilson quietly said, "Honey, I saw Jesus sitting here with us during the prayer…"

As a wave of peace came over me, I was able to visualize Jesus at his bedside. Then these words came to my mind: "I rise from the waters to declare that Jesus walked with me every step of the way."

As much as I hated the situation we were in, I was comforted knowing that Jesus was at Wilson's side. I spent the night watching him fall in and out of sleep while I madly put together the order of service for his Celebration of Life. When Wilson awoke the next morning, I shared with him what would be most of my eulogy. We went through some photos and videos of our children on my computer before I went home to spend a few hours with the twins.

When Rose left, I was overcome with sadness. I rethought my farewell party. I was really tired. I was tired of fighting. I couldn't stand living with this pain any longer. Why was I prolonging the inevitable? I couldn't wait for Thursday.

Tonight will be my last night. Lord, I am ready to come home.

As I left the hospital, I desperately wanted to hold on to Wilson. I dreaded the thought that I wouldn't be able to hear his voice, feel the warmth of his hands and know that I was truly loved. And as much I dreaded the pain and suffering that I would endure in facing a life without my soulmate, I saw that the man lying in the hospital bed before me was suffering—mentally and physically. It is in our suffering that we draw undeniably closer to God.

It was in this moment that God asked the both of us to reflect on our time these forty-plus days in the hospital. We had asked God for more time. He had given us an extra four weeks. In those four weeks, we both grew closer to Him, especially Wilson. His faith and trust in Him grew in leaps and bounds. We were jumping off cliffs for God. God allowed Wilson's parents to be witnesses to the power of prayer and gave Wilson opportunities to share his faith and his testimony with his family and staff in the hospital.

God calmed our hearts and reminded us that He gave Wilson thirty-five years after his fall in Thailand, eight years since almost falling off a cliff, one and a half years after his tumour hemorrhaged and, most recently, an extra six weeks in the hospital after his first intestinal blockage.

God is merciful and gracious. We are not meant to live forever on Earth. The goal of this life is to meet God in our suffering and to understand our true purpose.

Wilson will always be the love of my life, my hero and my fighter. He always stood up for the right thing and was persistent in pursuing his goals. I knew that he had been fighting this battle with cancer for me and for the twins. He wanted to share more of himself with them. He wanted to be there to celebrate their successes and to mentor them through life's challenges. Above all else, he wanted to show them how much he loved them.

When I returned to the hospital later that morning, Wilson said to me, "Rose, I can't wait for Thursday. It's too hard. It has to be tonight."

I understood in my self-reflection, prompted by the Spirit, that Wilson needed me to tell him it was okay—okay for him to stop fighting. So I said, "I love you. Don't worry, I will be okay. We will be okay. I will go home to get the twins. I will let everyone know our change in plans. Tonight will be your last night."

I quickly contacted a few of his friends to pass on the message that Thursday's party was cancelled and that if they wanted to see Wilson, they would have to come to the hospital today.

As I was getting the twins, I also grabbed a copy of our wedding vows. I had my sister record our last family moment with Wilson explaining how much he loved each of them and that he had to go home to be with Jesus. We had preplanned what we would say to the twins about "Daddy's absence," a message based on John 14: 1–4 (NKJV):

> Let not your heart be troubled: you believe in God, believe also in me. In my Father's house are many mansions: if it were not so, I would have told you. I go to prepare a place for you. And if I go and prepare a place for you, I will come again and receive you to myself; that where I am, there you may be also. And where I go you know, and the way you know.

We explained that Daddy would head to Heaven first to build our home and prepare our rooms. We would see him again when God called us home. The twins had just turned three. It was obvious to them that their beloved daddy was sick. Most of our videos, prayers and conversations up until this point had centred around Daddy coming home to our house, not God's. In truth, I am not sure how much they understood.

In the hospital room, they listened, and they scurried around Daddy asking questions about the tubes he had coming off his body. They understood that this would be the last time they saw him. Together, we reinforced how Daddy would be heading to a place with God, where he would receive a new body and endure no pain or suffering.

After this family moment, I had my brother-in-law record Wilson and me as we renewed our wedding vows. I wanted to remind Wilson that I never regretted marrying him. Many people walk through life never finding someone to share their life with, let alone meet someone who can read their thoughts and make them feel loved unconditionally. A few close friends referred to us as "an old married couple." How fitting, foreshadowing our expedited timeline. Although God planned that we wouldn't make it past our fourteenth anniversary, we lived and loved like we had just celebrated our fiftieth.

That Tuesday was a blur. Wilson's friends and extended family members came in droves to visit him late that afternoon. We had a lineup of people for at least three hours. I became an usher. I met people in the hallway and directed them into the room. They offered their condolences and hugs. It was a sad day for all of us.

In truth, it was a crazy day. All I can say is that God stood behind me and lifted me up. He gave me the strength I needed to push through for Wilson. I refrained from getting too emotionally wrapped up in what was occurring. I limited each visit to about five to seven minutes, just so I could usher in the next group.

About an hour into the visits, I found myself at Wilson's bedside, helping his friends to hear him, because he had lost his voice. He smiled for each guest, despite his physical pain, and still warmly congratulated his friends who were pregnant. We even had a nurse from our previous ward come and visit him, for she was touched by Wilson's courage and love for God.

By eight o'clock, Wilson told me he was done seeing guests. The last guests he saw were his nephew, who had flown in from Toronto, and his two friends from high school. After his final guests left, just after eight thirty, Wilson turned to me and said, "I'm done, Rose. I have nothing left to say to you. I have said all I needed to say. I'm really tired. Please make sure I don't wake up."

Wilson officially passed away at 5:55 p.m. on Saturday, March 25, 2017, four days after he said his official goodbyes to everyone.

15

Reflection of God's Love
(from Rose's perspective)

I remember leaving the hospital that last night with the distinct smell of Wilson on my body and in my mind—a reminder that I would no longer see or embrace his physical body. He wished to be cremated, and his remains were to be scattered into the ocean. The next day was Sunday. I tried to run things 'business as usual' for the benefit of the twins, but as I was dressing them for church, I smelled that same distinct scent of Wilson as I was walking in the hallway of my home! I literally stopped in my tracks.

I couldn't help but smile. I felt Wilson all around me. I knew his heart was burdened and guilt-laden for not just leaving me, but also for leaving me to raise the twins on my own. I felt Wilson's presence with me at church that morning too. I felt him sitting next to me, asking me to lean into him while we sat together in the pew.

I hesitated to tell this to others, especially those who weren't spiritual. I feared being judged and called crazy. I couldn't blame them—I may have thought and said the same thing. But there was no denying what I felt. Just as the risen Christ appeared to Thomas, so was this presence of Wilson to me.

As much as people tried to be helpful, I could not ask them to shoulder the burden of certain things alongside me. One of these was clearing out Wilson's belongings—his clothes, his gadgets, his mail. Each item of his triggered a memory, which led to a tidal wave of emotions that swept over me. The subsequent pain likened to daggers piercing my heart deeper and deeper. But as stressed, sad and dejected as I felt, I recognized that I had nothing to fear. Wilson was exactly where he needed to be. Home—his final home. Knowing he was with God provided me with the comfort I needed to move forward.

I realized how blessed I was to be present for Wilson as his disease progressed and his symptoms unfolded—not only to care for him, but to witness his faith blossom. As hard as I had tried to get Wilson to commit to God in our years together, I had failed each time. But God was always in the background, waiting. He had equipped us with all that we had needed.

While Wilson was bedridden, he was driven to spend time with God. In addition to my daily devotional readings and prayers, Wilson also spent time willingly listening to sermons online or watching video enactments of Biblical stories. It was clear to me that God was taking time to purify him as in Psalm 119 where we are reminded that God's word is the lamp unto our feet. He was letting Wilson be trampled on, to remind him to keep his eye on the prize—God Himself.

Wilson left me with many gifts. What I valued most was his complete trust, love and loyalty. He was intent on ensuring that I knew he loved me. In fact, I knew he couldn't love me any more than he did. For more than two years, he made it a point to tell me that he loved me at least once a day. I can still hear him tell me, "You are the best thing that happened to me, then the kids. I love all of you." What I didn't realize was that most people at his workplace also knew how much he loved me. He would beam while talking about me to his co-workers.

Wilson had great qualities, and some not-so-great ones too. One of his friends fondly reminisced,

> Wilson could be forgetful at times. I still remember the time when he left his laptop bag in the parking lot and accidently ran over it with his car. I loved how he was able to make light of the situation and was still able to laugh about his mistake.

It was evident how much Wilson grew to love the Lord. However, there were seasons in his life when God fell to the background. In truth, I would describe Wilson's faith like a roller coaster ride. He was up and then down, hot and then cold. At one point, God even ended up on his 'hate' list! Then there were seasons when Wilson cried out to Him in thanksgiving and in pain.

Wilson commonly recited and sang Pete Seeger's "Turn! Turn! Turn!," a song based on verses from the book of Ecclesiastes. He recognized how precious time is and the importance of seizing opportunities to live fully and righteously. There is an appropriate time for everything. We have no control over when we are born or when we die, experience extreme pain or love.

Wilson's faith reflected his personality. For when he was thirsty for anything, he drank his fill—filled his cup until it was overflowing. Then he'd stop for a season and repeat the process by overindulging. This behaviour was not unique to Wilson, for many of us fear and believe that God may not be there to catch us when we fall.

While Wilson was undergoing cancer treatment, I often thought of Job. I saw how Job's faith was tested, and I used Job's faith as a personal benchmark. After the Lord took away Job's wealth, his children and even his health, Job still refused to deny God's love for him and continued to praise Him. From Job 1:21 (NIV),

> Then Job fell to the ground in worship and said, "Naked I came from my mother's womb, and naked I will depart. The Lord gave and the Lord has taken away; may the name of the Lord be praised."

While Wilson was sick, I saw him play the role of Job. In Job's story, there was a happy ending. I kept hoping for the same for Wilson. I hoped that God would restore Wilson to full strength in this world. Yet, as Wilson's body started failing him, this passage came to mind, Philippians 1:21(NIV): "For to me, to live is Christ and to die is gain."

My crutch in this life, the love of my life, was taken from me. Yet contrary to what people expected, I wasn't angry with God. What I felt instead was awe. I felt blessed to have been loved by a man whose love was enough to last many lifetimes over. God knew Wilson would die from cancer. Yes, God allowed Wilson to die relatively young. But every living thing on this earth will eventually die and wither away. We are all "candles in the wind." We just don't know how and when our light will be blown out.

God showed me that Wilson left this world just as he had come into it—with a bang. Wilson lived his life well. He worked hard to provide for his family, but he also took time to fully enjoy things like food, entertainment and spending time with friends. He spoke his mind and was mindful about helping others. In particular, he regularly bought meals for the homeless.

One of God's greatest gifts to me was giving me the privilege of raising two 'mini-Wilsons'. It is no coincidence that friends who knew Wilson immediately recognize how both twins exemplify some of his characteristics. I can already see that Isaac has inherited his father's sense of curiosity, joking nature, loyalty and sense of justice. As for Bella, she has Wilson's profound love for fun and care for family.

I have found solace in choosing to remember and celebrate Isaac and Isabella's beloved daddy and honour his memory every Christmas, birthday and Father's Day by going through a photo album and a few family videos. I hope that by routinely bringing up Wilson, I can help them get to know their father through my eyes. My daily bedtime prayer ends with this phrase to remind them how much they are loved, "Mommy loves you. Daddy loves you. God loves you. Jesus loves you."

In his journey home to God, Wilson left a great impression on those who knew him and definitely made this world a little better than he had found it.

Afterword

God prepared me well for this role of being a widow and sole parent left behind. God reminded me on several occasions that "He has prepared me for such a time as this." So when people wonder how I can appear so 'normal', I tell them that I have learned to accept that every day is a gift. I choose to live accordingly for the sake of my children and God. My job on Earth is not done. Life is a wonderful and priceless gift. As homage to God, we should take advantage of the opportunities He gives us to serve Him by loving others as He loves us.

Writing this book has helped me see God in a new light. I see how He has been consistently present in my life without needing to shout. In my first year of grief and loss, God gifted me with a series of visions to comfort me in the loss of my husband, closest friend and confidant.

God didn't speak to me in my dreams, instead he ensured that I was awake and fully conscious. First, He showed me a vision of infinite lights in a dark room. As my eyes adjusted and accepted the wondrous beauty of the lights, I began to take notice as they randomly burned out. God was telling me that behind every light was a story—each one of significance. Some stories were more painful or heroic than others, but each was special in its own way.

I soon began to wonder why I was unable to see what happened to the lights after they were gone. God then reminded me that light is energy. As dictated by the laws of science, energy cannot be created or destroyed, just displaced. We are those lights. Those are our stories. Those are our lives. Each light represents our souls.

God also asked me to see this life from the perspective of being 'in transit'. Our present life is synonymous with being at a train station we all arrive, and we all depart. But it is the choices we make in this life that determine which train we will board. I know Wilson is safe with Christ in Heaven, and that's the train I will board one day in the future too. My task is to make sure that all the people I love also end up on this Heaven-bound train.

I recognize that although an amazing chapter of my life has ended, God is leading me into a new one. From Psalm 139:16 (NIV): "Your eyes saw my unformed body; all the days ordained for me were written in your book before one of them came to be."

God knows everything, as He is the author and director of my life story. At times, I thought His hand was absent, but He has proven to me time and time again that He is observing us close by. One of his final images to me was of a dove carrying a ribbon or branch. He is promising me peace and freedom. I can hear Him saying, "Rose, embrace your new beginning and follow me."

Appendix A: Letters to Isaac and Isabella

Dear Isaac and Isabella,

By the time you are able to read this letter, you probably want to know more about your daddy. I made a promise to him that I'd try my best to give you a glimpse of what kind of a person he was.

To give you some background, I worked with your daddy from 2010 until 2012. It wasn't a long time that we worked together, but he was an important person to me, and I have always considered him my mentor. Without his guidance, I'm not sure if I would be where I am today. He was the senior manager, and this was my first project management job. I wanted to quit and really questioned my value at the company. But your daddy was always there to give me great advice.

When we had bad days, we would go to the local Starbucks to vent (and we were there a lot). He usually started with his favourite tag line, "You buying?" Then he'd follow with, "A tall Americano in a grande cup!"

Don't get me wrong; he was a generous man, but he enjoyed harassing us to buy him coffee. In fact, he was often the one who bought us coffee and lunches and was kind enough to do the same to those he didn't even know. He had a great sense of humour and was always doing what was right. Sometimes, doing what was right didn't align with what the company wanted. But Wilson would fight for what was in the best interest of the customer.

He loved your mommy very much, and it really showed whenever he talked about her. I still remember the time when we went on a business trip to Edmonton. He deliberately chose to stay at the Fantasyland Hotel in West Edmonton Mall because he said the last time he was there was with your mommy, at least a decade earlier. This hotel was far from our project site and clearly outdated. There were better hotels to stay at, but he chose this hotel to reminisce about the time he spent there with your mom. Although he didn't always say the sweetest things, his actions clearly showed how much he loved her.

I still remember how happy he was when he found out he was going to be a father. When you two were born, he told me how much joy you both brought, and he urged me to become a parent of my own child someday. He not only gave me great advice professionally, but he was a good friend who gave me advice in other parts of my life. I am very thankful that I had a chance to know him. Seeing all the people who came to say goodbye to him at the hospital showed how many people's lives he touched and how much we all loved him.

From what I know, your daddy wants you to both be happy and healthy and to be kind to those around you. He made a positive impact on those who knew him, and I am blessed to have these memories of him. He genuinely cared for all around him, and I know he will be looking down from heaven, protecting you all.

Lots of love, and God bless.

A friend of your daddy's
Vancouver, BC, Canada
April 2017

Dearest Isabella and Isaac,

I hope this letter finds you both when you are a bit older and can give you a tiny glimpse of what your daddy was like. He touched so many lives and made this world a brighter and friendlier place. I hope you guys will continue his legacy of sharing laughter and kindness with those you meet in the magical journey called life.

I am thankful that I knew Wilson and have shared a good chuckle with him. I wanted to share a few memories of Wilson with you both.

Your daddy was quite the jokester. We were on a four-member team business trip in Juneau, Alaska. Your daddy was our project manager. Because we were travelling during the off-season, the team had very few options for accommodations. We ended up staying at Grandma's Feather Bed—isn't that a ridiculous name? The decor of the place was of a doll house. Your daddy stayed in a room that had baby pink walls and big white doll-like furniture. The whole time we were there, your daddy would joke around and tell the team how the hotel was haunted by "Granny." He would have the team guess which room was Granny's. Although we missed home, trips with your daddy were always eventful.

During dinner, at a random Chinese restaurant in Alaska, your daddy pulled out his wallet and showed us a small photo of your mom and him when they were younger. This was before the time of smartphones with built-in digital cameras. It was so sweet. We could tell how much your daddy loved your mommy.

Your daddy was a funny man, but he also had a big heart. He eagerly offered to help whoever needed support. When I told him I left the company that we both worked at and was in the market for a new job, without a blink of the eye, he asked if he could help me. He was so kind and offered to be my reference and also passed on my information to people who he felt might be interested in my skill set.

Another time, I mentioned to your daddy that I was building a house. Without hesitation, he invited me over to see if he could help with design or building questions. That same day, your daddy gave my husband and me a tour of your home and shared his experiences in the hopes of helping us avoid any pitfalls in our own house project. On the tour, when we reached the nursery, I originally declined to look inside, in fear of waking two sweet babies peacefully sleeping. The babies were none other than you guys! But your daddy, the proud and loving father he was, encouraged us to peek inside as he was excited for us to see you. He beamed with love. You both were such gifts to your daddy. He loved you with all his being.

Your daddy was truly a wonderfully kind, funny and generous human. I feel lucky to have known your daddy. My heart continues to weep knowing that his physical body is no longer with us. But I take comfort that I have these memories and can share some with you.

The maternal side of me wishes for you both to live a colourful life with no regrets, to be compassionate to yourselves and others, share laughter and spread love wherever you both may go in this lifetime. I'm sure your daddy would want the same.

Peace, love and rainbows of light, precious little gems.

A friend of your daddy's
Vancouver, BC, Canada
April 2017

Appendix B: Testimonials

Wilson's friends and family also saw his sense of loyalty, courage and humility. Here are testimonials from his best friend from high school and from his brother-in-law.

******

Wilson and I first met through a mutual friend, Daniel. Wilson was one of the five guys in our group, and we all hung out together during lunch hour or after school. I feel we didn't get along well because I was new. It felt like Wilson was sizing me up; he was very standoffish. One of my favourite memories of Wilson is when Daniel, Wilson and I skipped class and instead went to a Japanese restaurant where we ordered sushi for the first time. Wilson went to the washroom, and while he was gone, Daniel and I decided to trick him. We told him to eat the entire green mushy blob to cleanse his taste buds. He started crying and spit out the wasabi before downing multiple glasses of water. From that moment on, Wilson and I began to spend more time together. Wilson really warmed up to me when he learned my father had died when I was young and that my brother was someone with special needs. I felt accepted and understood.

One day in grade nine, Wilson found me in one of the halls at school and asked me to work out with him in the weight room. I was very reluctant. I was already a pretty big guy, and the last thing I wanted to do was get muscular. But he convinced me to join him, and we worked out every lunch hour and every day after school. We were getting to be good friends. Then came summer and the two of us started hanging out even more. On the weekends, we would often go to the movies and then to dinner after. We would watch one movie and then sneak into a different theatre in the same complex to watch another. We also got really into martial arts movies like *Bloodsport* and *Kickboxer*. One time, Wilson and I decided to learn to do the splits like Jean-Claude van Damme. I remember we would fool around the gym doing splits and karate kicks in between our weightlifting sets. We were always trying to outdo each other.

In grade ten, I got asked to join the rugby team. Wilson convinced me to give up badminton and play on the team with him. We were like brothers. He had my back and I had his.

It was also around this time that Wilson started to drift away from Daniel and the rest of the guys. The guys all started to tease him and make fun of him. I saw less of Wilson during lunch, but still I'd see him in the gym after school.

"I'm a nerd and I like nerds," I recall him saying one day. I think it was grade eleven. He had either made a realization or had been hit in the head too hard. Wilson started talking about these girls in school that he was crushing on. He started hanging out with other kids in school. I still hung out with Daniel and our crew, and they started to forget about Wilson. It bothered Wilson and I think he wrote a poem that was put into a yearbook.

I believe it was also in grade eleven when Wilson got his licence and access to a car. This began the late-night drives on which I would learn of his love of '80s love songs and his lack of fear to sing out loud. He would share about girls he liked, cars and poems that he wrote. Also, there was a night he confessed he never liked me at first and always wanted to fight me. We still did our movies and dinners, but we didn't have to bus or SkyTrain home after. We went to Chinese double features; the first movie would be an action movie, and the second feature was always something Rrated. We were boys and the raging hormones were starting.

Wilson was family. He was my brother. He would charm my mom and my sister by telling them how good they looked. He would joke with my brother. On Sundays, I would be getting dropped off from church, and I'd see his car parked outside my house. He would be waiting for me to get home. I decided to invite him out to fellowship one Friday night. I swear, if a person was female and had legs, there would be Wilson trying to charm them to their knees. I have never seen someone flirt so much. Everyone loved him.

— *From Steve Ng, Wilson's best friend
from high school and best man at Wilson
and Rose's wedding.*

Wilson had a strong sense of protectiveness for his sister. In a way, I had to prove myself. It wasn't about demonstrating status or wealth, but rather building on one of the values that Wilson valued most—loyalty. Loyalty and trust are strongly related; both take time and effort to build and maintain, and both can be destroyed with one act in an instant. Wilson was fiercely protective of those that he cared for—his family, his friends, his teammates and his colleagues.

I came to fully appreciate Wilson's sense of loyalty when I had the privilege of working with him at Wolf Medical. We had both been recruited to build superior capabilities on Wolf's operations teams, but he had the added responsibility of nurturing a high-performing engineering team under intense delivery demands. Wilson had a simple but powerful strategy: hire highly capable people, set clear expectations for their performance and then stand back and let them work.

He had one simple rule that I continue to use to this day: he would tell his team that he trusted them to get the job done and that if they screwed up, he'd have their backs as long as they were honest with him. "I will always have your back as long as you're straight with me," he would tell them. Wilson understood that trust and loyalty were the foundations of strong and lasting relationships, and this was one of the things I most valued in the relationship I eventually developed with him.

I met Wilson when he was really hitting his stride in terms of his career and enjoying the rewards of his efforts. I came to know that, early in his career, the company he worked for was actively recruiting for project managers for high-profile medical imaging deployment projects and gave internal team members a chance to apply. Although trained as an engineer and lacking any project management experience, Wilson saw the potential that this opportunity presented to advance his career and applied for the role. His drive and commitment won the confidence of his managers, and with a crash course and Project Management Professional (PMP) designation, he was soon running multi-million-dollar projects across the United States.

A project manager has a lot of responsibility and accountability but almost no direct authority and must rely as much on exceptional interpersonal and persuasive ability as good organization and planning skills. Wilson consistently exceeded delivery expectations and was rewarded handsomely for doing so. He liked his cars, he liked his vacations, he liked his watches and his pet fish. He worked hard, he played hard. He'd decide on a whim to drive down to Oregon for a night, enjoying a nice steak dinner and dune buggy adventures along the way with his wife, Rose, and whoever else wanted to share in the adventure. He often paid for dinners with family and friends, always generous and quick to share his good fortune with those he cared about.

When he was recruited for Wolf, it was a chance to build a high-performing team from scratch, a bigger challenge that carried significant risk and required him to give up the security he had built at his previous job with McKesson. I saw first-hand how much he contributed to the remarkable growth and success of the company, though he wouldn't talk about himself that way. It was a scary time for many of us; the growth was happening so fast that everything felt just slightly out of control, all of the time. Our projects relied on government funding and scrutiny. Our product had all kinds of bugs and glitches, and our teams were small and stretched thin. Wilson had a knack of knowing when the teams were particularly run ragged. Often he'd round up the whole group for lunch, demonstrating appreciation and a steady hand in rough waters, which I know helped keep the team pulling in the same direction.

As far as vices go, Wilson was pretty 'straight and narrow', but he had a taste for gambling. Poker was his game of choice, and I think he enjoyed just about any opportunity to play. He'd get together with buddies for poker night and jump at a chance to hit the casino with family members, or he would play by himself online.

Generally, Wilson was a fairly open book. I would characterize him as a poor liar, but he had a good 'poker face' and was skilled enough that he won more than he lost. It was one of the few things that he was more guarded about. And while I don't believe he ever outright hid his casino visits or online activities, he may have underplayed them a bit. It certainly wasn't anything that ever impacted his relationship or his financial well-being. From what I could gather, he'd keep his winnings set aside so he could continue gambling relatively risk- and guilt-free.

I suspect that Wilson had a particular talent for poker that might have led to greater financial gain had he seriously pursued it. I think he also understood that it could become a more dangerous addiction with more serious consequences. So he found a balance, kept it in check and found a way to 'scratch the itch' without letting it control him.

Meeting Rose was something Wilson deeply treasured, and he didn't want to lose her. I think it was a number of these defining moments in Wilson's life that slowly diffused the anger and the temper and led him to be the kind of guy that can joke and tease and poke fun at his friends and family and himself with equal ease. For me, real friendship is established when you can get past the egos and be able to tease and poke fun at each other. A connection is meaningful when we can get below the surface and when we can both admit that we're just happy fools that are lucky to be sharing some time together on this earth. There are not many people that I would say I have that connection with, but I'm glad to have had it with Wilson.

Ultimately, I think that Wilson's courage gave him wonderful opportunities and quality of life. Humility allowed him to find meaning and to live a fulfilling life. His loyalty gave him a loving family and friends for life.

— From John Weger
Wilson's brother-in-law

Acknowledgements

The completion of this legacy book project for my children would not have been possible without support from all members of Wilson's family—especially his parents and siblings, who shared their different perspective stories about coming to Canada. Equally important were friends who shared how Wilson impacted their lives and those who spent time babysitting my twins so I could devote time to writing my manuscript.

Finally, thank you, God, for giving me the strength and ability to bring this book to fruition. You remind me time and time again that as long as I walk with You, nothing is impossible. This process not only allowed me fully to grieve and feel the gravity of my loss, but more importantly also allowed me to cherish and relive my life knowing that I was blessed with a caring, loving and supportive husband, Wilson Ngo.